Eat Well! Cook Well!

The
BUSY MOM'S
COOKBOOK

The
BUSY MOM'S
COOKBOOK

100 RECIPES FOR QUICK, DELICIOUS, HOME-COOKED MEALS

ANTONIA LOFASO

with

CANDICE L. DAVIS

AVERY
a member of Penguin Group (USA) Inc.
New York

Published by the Penguin Group
Penguin Group (USA) Inc., 375 Hudson Street,
New York, New York 10014, USA

USA · Canada · UK · Ireland · Australia
New Zealand · India · South Africa · China

Penguin Books Ltd, Registered Offices: 80 Strand, London WC2R 0RL, England
For more information about the Penguin Group visit penguin.com

Most Avery books are available at special quantity discounts for bulk purchase for sales promotions, premiums, fund-
raising, and educational needs. Special books or book excerpts also can be created to fit specific needs. For details,
write: Special.Markets@us.penguingroup.com

Library of Congress Cataloging-in-Publication Data

Lofaso, Antonia.
The busy mom's cookbook : 100 recipes for quick, delicious, home-cooked meals / Antonia Lofaso ;
with Candice L. Davis.
p.   cm.
Includes index.
ISBN 978-1-58333-470-6
1. Cooking.   I. Davis, Candice L.   II. Title.
TX714.L637   2012   2012014583
641.3—dc23

ISBN 978-1-58333-533-8 (paperback edition)

Printed in the United States of America
3 5 7 9 10 8 6 4 2

BOOK DESIGN BY TANYA MAIBORODA

The recipes contained in this book are to be followed exactly as written. The publisher is not responsible for your specific
health or allergy needs that may require medical supervision. The publisher is not responsible for any adverse reactions
to the recipes contained in this book.

ALWAYS LEARNING   PEARSON

To Xea, who makes the occasional craziness

of the busy mom lifestyle worth every minute—

as I pursue my passion,

you're my greatest inspiration.

And to all the other busy moms trying to balance it all—

just remember none of us can pull this off alone.

We're all in it together.

CONTENTS

WELCOME TO THE BUSY MOM'S TABLE

Ever found yourself sprinting through the grocery store at seven o'clock in the morning, hoping you'll find something better than shrink-wrapped cheese and crackers to pack for lunch? When your son signs you up to make two dozen cookies for the school bake sale, do your thoughts immediately turn to slice and bake? Are you now, or have you ever been, on a first-name basis with every delivery dude from the local pizza place, and have you ever found yourself peeking out the window and hoping it's the hot guy this time?

Whether you're a single mom like me, a stay-at-home mom, a mom with a demanding job outside the house, or some combination of all of those, there's one thing we all have in common: we're busy! The recipes and tips in this book were designed to help bring the family together for meals, even as you juggle that busy lifestyle. At the end of the day, it doesn't matter if your experience of family is a mom and her preschooler coloring pictures and telling knock-knock jokes while they eat or a rowdy gathering of parents and kids, aunties and uncles, grandparents and best friends fiercely debating which team will win the next big game. It's all family, and it's time to gather our families around the table again.

FOOD AND FAMILY

It could've been Rice-A-Roni with scrambled eggs, or a big dinner I helped my mom or my dad make. Either way, it was very important to my parents that we all sit together and share meals when I was growing up. They demonstrated to me how people learn about family and community through food. People bond over food. Good food makes people happy!

Growing up in a traditional Italian-American household meant I was always surrounded by food and family. The two were inseparable for us. Food was one of the ways we took care of one another and shared our love. And it was meant to be shared with everyone. If the cable guy came to the house, my dad would make him a sandwich. Cooking was a natural part of life and experimenting in the kitchen was one of my favorite ways to spend my free time.

I always knew I wanted to be a chef. I just wasn't sure it was a possibility for me. It seemed like the type of career people dream of but few actually ever succeed at—like becoming an actor or an artist. It wasn't until my daughter Xea's dad, Dwight, asked me what I really loved to do that I started to think it might be possible to make a living doing a job I enjoyed. As I look back, it seems crazy that I thought working and doing what you love didn't go together.

By the time I decided to go to culinary school, I was waiting tables and pregnant with Xea. It was a serious struggle, but with help from family, especially Xea's grandparents, I graduated from the French Culinary Institute in New York City. The most important lesson I learned during that period of my life is that the all-powerful supermom who does it all by herself is just a myth. We all need help, especially as we try to balance work and parenthood.

Right after graduation, I had the opportunity to work at Spago, back in Los Angeles. Although the pay was low and the hours were long, I jumped at the opportunity. Friends thought I was crazy, that I was wasting my time in the job, but I saw it as an opportunity to learn from some of the best in the restaurant business. I was making only seven dollars an hour, but I was gaining a wealth of experience. Early on, I figured out I'd have to be incredibly organized to balance the demanding job with raising Xea.

Seven years later, I secured my first position as executive chef. While I was planning the menu for the new restaurant, I was offered the opportunity to audition for *Top Chef: Chicago*. I had never thought of doing a television show, but when I made it through the audition process, I knew I had to commit 100 percent. Leaving Xea for an undetermined amount of time, knowing I'd be able to call home only once in a while, was incredibly hard, of course. Even though she was with her dad, I was used to being there to control and oversee all the details of her day, and letting go of that was a challenge.

But letting go was the only way I'd have a chance to succeed on the show. On previous seasons of *Top Chef*, I'd seen too many chefs crying about missing their kids, then getting eliminated in the same episode. I didn't want Xea to ever think that a few weeks apart would make or break our relationship. Instead, I wanted her to see her mom as focused and ambitious and great at what I do. I let that motivate me to make it to the finals.

Since I competed on *Top Chef*, so many new opportunities have opened up for me. The most amazing result of being on the show is that I now run into people all over the country who want to experience my cooking. They relate to my story and they've seen how passionate I am about food. It's such a privilege to have that kind of support; without the show, it would've taken years to build this kind of career.

With all its benefits, the demands of my profession have also meant asking my daughter to master some of the skills of self-sufficiency. While we have a tremendous network of family support, Xea has also stepped up to the challenge. Sometimes that means she packs her own lunch, makes the crepes for our breakfast, or accompanies me to work at a charity event. I may not be home for dinner, but we have breakfast together every day, and when I'm traveling, we rely on technology to keep in touch.

I'm not willing to sacrifice my career or my role as a mom, so I work hard to balance the two. I can't say it's always easy. It's a work in progress, and as our situation changes, we adjust. Xea recently lost her father, which has presented a whole new set of challenges. Fortunately, our mother-daughter relationship is strong and our lives continue to be filled with loving and supportive friends and family. If I can't be there to sit at the dinner table with her, I don't have to worry. She's always breaking bread with someone who loves her, even if it's not me.

The Busy Mom's Cookbook is about bringing people back to that family meal as a means of giving one another undivided attention. It's about giving parents a way to pass on their heritage to their children, the way my parents and grandparents did for me and I'm doing for my daughter. Many women (and men, too) are convinced they can't teach their kids about food because they're not professional chefs, they didn't learn to cook from their mothers, and they don't have hours to spend in the kitchen. It's not about formal training, and it's not about the quantity of time you spend sweating over the stove. It's about the quality of the relationship when you share the experience of making and eating real food with your kids.

SEVEN TRUTHS ABOUT THE BUSY MOM

1. **We are, first and foremost, moms.** We meet with teachers, wipe runny noses, remind little ones that showering should actually be a daily occurrence, and occasionally show up for a meeting with peanut butter on our sleeve. It's who we are.

2. **We're more than just moms.** Our kids are top priority, but we still have our own careers, interests, passions, relationships, hobbies, pursuits, and dreams. While raising my daughter, Xea, I've completed culinary school, honed my craft under some of the most respected chefs in the business, competed twice on Bravo's *Top Chef*, and dedicated a year to planning and opening a new restaurant—with lots of help, of course!

3. **One parent plus one child equals a family.** A family is a family, whether it's two people or twelve. Single parents, two parents, blended families—it doesn't matter. Two people at the table are all you need for a family meal.

4. **There's no such thing as perfect balance in our lives.** It's a daily juggling act, and we get better at it by planning, organizing, and asking for help. The more we practice those skills, the easier it gets to keep all those balls marked career, kids, friends, family, and fun in the air. Still, we couldn't do it without help from our children's fathers, grandparents, and aunties and uncles, and from our friends, neighbors, and coworkers—anyone who's part of the team that helps us get things done and maintain sanity. We need the community we cobble together. It really does take a village!

5. **Sometimes, what we need is a kid-free moment.** We wouldn't be human if we didn't occasionally crave time alone or a few hours among adults. I say, eat at home more often, and use the money you would've spent dining out for a trip to the spa!

6. **We get tired.** Duh! We're taking on a lot, and even with help, it would be crazy to think we don't get worn out sometimes.

7. **Even when we get tired, we get up and keep going.** Wouldn't it be nice to spend the day in bed with a bucket of ice cream, or a tub of cookie dough, and the remote control? Let somebody else make breakfast, mop the kitchen floor, and type up that overdue book report. Uh, not gonna happen.

Those are simple truths about being a modern mother. It doesn't matter if you're a stay-at-home mom, a working single mom, or a mother and wife and small-business owner. We're always balancing our needs with those of the people we love most in the world. Read on for seven rules that can help make home-cooked, family-centered meals a valuable part of that equation.

SEVEN RULES FOR THE BUSY MOM'S KITCHEN

1. **Start off small.** If you cook only on Thanksgiving and Christmas, and your culinary contribution usually consists of opening a can of biscuits, don't wake up the day after you get *The Busy Mom's Cookbook* and try to commit to a month of homemade meals. After a week or so of trying a new dish each day, you'd be ready to practice everything you learned in your kickboxing class on the next person who asked you what you're making for dinner. Start off with one extra home-cooked meal the first week. Next week, plan for two more than you'd usually make, and build from there. It gets easier with practice. Seriously.

2. **Speaking of planning . . . plan your menu a week or two ahead of time.** If you waited until the day of your daughter's soccer game to figure out how she'd get there, you'd probably end up with an unhappy kid on your hands, plus more chaos than necessary. Planning your schedule in advance makes life easier, gives kids a sense of stability, and preserves your sanity. So does planning meals. *The Busy Mom's Cookbook* will give you some ideas to make it easier to step back, take a deep breath, and plan it all out.

3. **Expect plans to change.** Kids get sick. Bosses ask us to stay at work an extra hour. Babysitters cancel at the last minute. It happens to the best of us. Be flexible, and roll with it.

4. **Sometimes you just have to serve the kids hot dogs, Stouffer's French bread pizza, or frozen waffles.** I do! I grew up eating that stuff once in a while, and I like it once in a while. You don't have to choose between feeding your kids and having a life. You're teaching your kids healthy living habits—everything in moderation.

5. **Let the kids in the kitchen—girls and boys.** Instead of wasting time and energy chasing them out, let them come in and peel a carrot or two. They'll feel like they've accomplished something, and they'll have learned new skills, which means they can help you more as they grow. The best part: you get to spend a few minutes talking with them without once saying do your homework, make your bed, or quit hitting your sister. Don't worry. There'll be plenty of time to nag later.

6. **Use the 15/15 Rule.** When there just doesn't seem to be enough time, spend fifteen minutes in the kitchen preparing a meal with your child and spend fifteen more seated at the table, sharing your meal. Take the time to look into his eyes, and ask him about his day. Get as much quality as you can out of it. Homework, the laundry, e-mail, and the season finale of whatever you're recording can wait for thirty minutes.

7. **Enjoy!** It's just food. I wrote this book to make life easier, not more complicated. I've included the full range of recipes—from fast and healthy meals both you and the kids will enjoy to slightly more involved, special recipes you can make for special occasions. They're recipes for real moms with real lives. No pressure.

I want *The Busy Mom's Cookbook* to be an inspiration to you, a busy, multitasking mom—a reminder to enjoy this part of family life. Big or small, every family deserves the sense of community that happens only when people break bread together. Many of our most intimate moments happen at the table. People get engaged and break up at the table. They announce promotions and straight-A report cards and celebrate every accomplishment over a shared meal. I hope this cookbook will remind you to slow down and enjoy one another. Experience a great meal with your child and create the kind of memories that happen only when you nourish each other with both fresh food and companionship. If your days are as busy as mine, trust me, your "to do" list will still be there.

THE BUSY MOM'S BASICS

When I moved away from home to go to college, I lived in a small apartment in New York City. It was my first place. I slept there and studied there, but I called my mom to complain that it just didn't feel like a home. She told me to go to the store and get some flour, sugar, and all the other baking essentials, along with a couple of boxes of pasta, some olive oil, and a few other things.

Once my kitchen was stocked, and I could jump in there and make myself a home-cooked meal, my apartment began to feel like home to me.

Here are some basics I suggest every mom have on hand to make quick meals and keep her house feeling like home.

Baking Supplies/Spices
all-purpose flour
baking powder
baking soda
Better Than Bouillon
black pepper
Cajun seasoning (any brand)
cinnamon
dried bread crumbs/panko
ground coriander
ground cumin
honey
dried Italian seasoning
lemon-pepper seasoning
light brown sugar
nutmeg
powdered sugar
salt
sugar
vanilla extract

Condiments
barbecue sauce
catsup
hot sauce
mayonnaise

oyster sauce
soy sauce
whole-grain and other mustards
Worcestershire sauce

Dairy and Eggs
block of Parmigiano-Reggiano
eggs
unsalted butter
whole milk

Oil and Vinegar
apple cider vinegar
balsamic vinegar
extra-virgin olive oil (for flavoring)
inexpensive olive oil (for cooking)
sherry vinegar
vegetable or canola oil

Pantry Staples
brown rice
canned beans
canned coconut milk, unsweentened
canned corn
canned crabmeat
canned kalamata olives

canned peaches
canned pineapple
canned tomatoes
canned tuna
capers
dried beans
parboiled rice
pasta (a few boxes)
premade tomato sauce
seasoned rice

Produce and Bread
bell peppers
butter lettuce
carrots
celery
fresh tomatoes
garlic
good-quality bread
lemons
limes
poultry mix of fresh herbs
   (rosemary, thyme,
   parsley, and oregano)
red and yellow onions
romaine lettuce

Breakfast and Brunch

LEMON CREPES

CREAMY POLENTA WITH MACERATED STONE FRUIT

FRESH STRAWBERRY-AND-MINT LIMEADE

OPEN-FACE BLT WITH EGGS ON THE SUNNY SIDE

CRISPY OLIVE OIL PANCAKES

RED BLISS POTATO AND SWEET ONION FRITTATA

BUTTERMILK BISCUITS WITH HONEY BUTTER

CAJUN COUNTRY POTATOES AND SAUSAGES

CRAB CAKES WITH CHIPOTLE ADOBO AIOLI

THE BEST BLUEBERRY MUFFINS

SMOKED SALMON WITH CRISPY POTATO PANCAKE

CUSTOMIZED MINI-FRITTATAS

CUCUMBER-WATERMELON SPRITZER WITH CHAMOMILE

THE FIRST TIME I EVER MADE BREAKFAST, I WAS FOUR YEARS OLD AND I THOUGHT it would be good to start with eggs. That's what my dad made us every day. So, on the one morning he overslept, I decided to handle it for him. My little brother sat in a corner of the kitchen playing with his Legos while I did the things I'd seen my dad do: crack the eggs, put them in the pan, throw the shells in the trash, and clean up.

My poor dad woke up in a panic, realizing he was late and thinking his kids must be starving. I kept trying to explain to him that I'd already started breakfast, but he was too busy searching for the egg pan to pay any attention to what the four-year-old was saying.

Finally I convinced him to check the oven. There he found the egg pan with three perfectly cracked and perfectly raw eggs sitting in it. I hadn't yet figured out that the oven actually had to be turned on. Oops.

My dad tells this little story all the time. He loves to brag that even as a small child, I kept a clean kitchen while I cooked, and I still do. I just love that we have this memory to share. It's one of hundreds of small moments that connect us.

Now that I have years of experience cooking for my own daughter, I've perfected some breakfast favorites. The recipes in this chapter will take you from busy workday mornings, when you're scrambling to get the kids out the door, to leisurely brunches when you can invite the kids to enjoy cooking with you and make your own kitchen memories.

Lemon Crepes

MAKES 12 crepes
TOTAL TIME: 15 minutes

This recipe is so simple that my eleven-year-old daughter makes it without my help. One day, she decided the powdered sugar and lemon juice should be blended together in a bowl and served like an icing. Feel free to steal her idea.

1¼ cups whole milk

4 medium or 3 large eggs

1¼ teaspoons vanilla extract

1¼ cups all-purpose flour

¼ teaspoon cinnamon

2 tablespoons sugar

¼ teaspoon salt

Nonstick vegetable oil spray, for pan

1 cup powdered sugar

3 lemons, quartered

WHAT TO DO

IN A BLENDER COMBINE the milk, eggs, and vanilla. Add the flour, cinnamon, sugar, and salt on top of the liquid ingredients. Blend for 25 to 30 seconds on high, just until incorporated. Be sure to add the wet ingredients to the blender first. If the dry ingredients go in first, the liquid won't reach the bottom and the flour will get caked under the blades.

SPRAY an 8-inch nonstick pan with nonstick spray and heat on medium. For each crepe, pour ¼ cup of batter in a very thin layer on the bottom of the pan. Cook for about 1½ minutes. The wetness will dissipate and the crepe will look like a very soft pancake.

FOLD the crepe in half to make a semicircle. Fold it in half again, so it's folded in fourths, forming a cone shape with one rounded end, and transfer it to a plate.

DUST the crepes generously with powdered sugar. Serve with a lemon quarter for each crepe. The lemons will be squeezed on top of each crepe and create a lemony icing as the juice mixes with the powdered sugar.

Creamy Polenta with Macerated Stone Fruit

SERVES 4
TOTAL TIME: 15 minutes

Maybe you've never thought of polenta as an option for breakfast, but this simple, warm dish makes a great replacement for the same old oatmeal or cold cereal. And kids love the sweetness of the fruit topping.

FOR THE POLENTA
8 cups whole milk
2 cups quick-cooking polenta

FOR THE FRUIT TOPPING
2 peaches, plums, or nectarines, pitted and sliced
¼ cup light brown sugar, firmly packed
¼ teaspoon salt
¼ teaspoon cinnamon, or 4 Microplane grates of a fresh cinnamon stick
¼ teaspoon nutmeg, or 4 Microplane grates of fresh nutmeg
Juice of one lemon

WHAT TO DO

IN A 4-QUART SAUCEPOT, heat the milk over medium heat until it reaches a simmer. Whisk in the polenta. It should be simmering, not boiling. Look for movement in the liquid and polenta, but if it's popping, reduce the heat to medium-low. Cook for 10 minutes, whisking every 2 minutes, and whisking again as it finishes cooking.

WHILE THE POLENTA COOKS, place the stone fruit in a medium bowl and toss it with the brown sugar, salt, cinnamon, nutmeg, and lemon juice. The brown sugar and salt will draw out the natural juices of the fruit, which will blend with the sugar to create a flavorful macerated fruit topping.

SERVE the polenta in four bowls, topping each with a spoonful of the fruit.

the
**BUSY
MOM'S
TIP**

If you can't find quick-cooking polenta, follow the package directions on whatever polenta your store has, but substitute water for the whole milk.

Fresh Strawberry-and-Mint Limeade

You'll get more juice from the strawberries if you juice them, but if you don't have a juicer, you can muddle them. Simply add them to the bottom of your pitcher and crush them with a spoon.

Don't forget that drinks offer another opportunity to be creative in the kitchen. This is a nice alternative to the usual lemonade and a fabulous alternative to soda, too. Your kids will love it.

4 cups water
Juice of 4 medium limes
2 cups strawberries, stemmed and juiced or muddled (see tip)
1 cup agave nectar
4 sprigs of mint, for garnish
8 berries, for garnish

WHAT TO DO

COMBINE the water, lime juice, strawberry juice, and agave nectar in a large pitcher and stir well. Serve over ice in four glasses and garnish with fresh mint and berries.

Open-Face BLT with
Eggs on the Sunny Side

This fork-and-knife sandwich goes great with a brunch Bloody Mary, or with the more kid-friendly Fresh Strawberry and Mint Limeade (page 14) or Cucumber-Watermelon Spritzer (page 32). I like your basic Oscar Mayer bacon, but you can also substitute turkey bacon, a speciality uncured bacon, or a vegetarian option, if you prefer. *(see photo insert)*

FOR THE SANDWICHES

1 pound bacon

2 (6-inch) baguettes, sliced lengthwise

4 large leaves butter lettuce (also known as Boston lettuce)

2 medium tomatoes, sliced

Salt to taste

Black pepper to taste

Nonstick vegetable oil spray or 2 tablespoons unsalted butter

4 large eggs

FOR THE TARRAGON MAYONNAISE

¼ cup mayonnaise

2 tablespoons chopped fresh tarragon (see tip) or 1½ teaspoons dried Italian seasoning (see tip, page 47)

Juice of ½ lemon

WHAT TO DO

COOK the bacon according to the package directions.

WHILE THE BACON IS COOKING, combine the mayonnaise, the tarragon, and the lemon juice in a small bowl and blend well.

SET THE BROILER to high and toast the baguette halves in the oven until they're slightly brown. It should take only about a minute.

the
**BUSY
MOM'S
TIP**

For the tarragon mayonnaise, you could also substitute 1½ tea-spoons dried tarragon for the fresh tarragon if you happen to have it on hand. Or you could swap the tarragon for another fresh herb.

SPREAD the tarragon mayonnaise on the toasted baguettes. Layer on the butter lettuce and tomato. Season the tomato with salt and pepper. Place the bacon on top.

SPRAY a 10-inch nonstick pan with nonstick vegetable oil spray, or melt 1 tablespoon of butter for each batch of eggs, and heat the pan on medium-low. You can make 2 sunny-side-up eggs at a time. Crack the eggs into the pan, keeping the heat low so the eggs don't brown. Cook the eggs for 3 to 5 minutes, or until both the yolks and the whites thicken and set. Layer 1 egg onto each sandwich and serve warm.

THE BUSY MOM'S COOKBOOK

Crispy Olive Oil Pancakes

Sunday-morning pancakes are my dad's specialty. This version is an homage to him and to his Italian heritage. Using olive oil instead of butter gives you a pancake that's crispier on the outside and still tender on the inside. If you're in the mood for something sweeter, try the chocolate pancake option.

2 cups all-purpose flour

½ cup sugar

2 tablespoons baking powder

1 teaspoon salt

Zest of 1 orange, finely chopped (optional)

1 cup buttermilk

2 cups whole milk

2 large eggs

4 teaspoons vanilla extract

2 tablespoons olive oil, plus extra for cooking

Blackberries and Devon cream, mascarpone cheese, or syrup, for serving
(optional)

WHAT TO DO

IN A MEDIUM BOWL, whisk together the flour, sugar, baking powder, salt, and zest, if using.

IN A SEPARATE BOWL, combine the buttermilk, milk, eggs, vanilla, and 2 tablespoons olive oil. Whisk well. Pour into the dry ingredient mixture and stir just until combined.

IN A LARGE NONSTICK PAN or on a flat griddle (see tip), heat 1½ tablespoons olive oil on medium-low. Do a test pancake to make sure the pan is hot enough. Use a 2-ounce ladle or ¼-cup measuring cup to portion your batter. When the pancakes

the
BUSY MOM'S TIP

A 24-inch griddle that covers two burners is great for larger families. They're not expensive and you can cook eight to ten pancakes at a time.

I used to keep the pancakes warm in the oven until the whole batch was done, but my dad insists they should be eaten hot from the pan. The larger griddle lets the whole family sit down to breakfast together.

have bubbles around the edges and in the center, they're ready to be flipped. They should take 1½ to 2 minutes on each side. Add 1½ tablespoons olive oil to the pan for each batch.

I LOVE TO SERVE these pancakes with blackberries and a drizzle of thick Devon cream or a little scoop of mascarpone cheese instead of butter. Any syrup you like is good, but maple syrup adds a richer flavor.

FOR CHOCOLATE PANCAKES

OMIT the zest and replace the 2 tablespoons olive oil with 2 tablespoons melted unsalted butter in the batter. Use nonstick vegetable oil spray instead of olive oil in your pan and add a sprinkle of semisweet chocolate chips to the pancakes while they're cooking on the first side.

Red Bliss Potato and
Sweet Onion Frittata

My mom gets credit for this dish. She'd make it for me when I was a kid and I would, on very rare occasions, pretend to be sick so I could stay home from school. It was her way of saying she knew I wasn't really sick and all I really needed was a little extra TLC.

5 tablespoons olive oil
½ medium yellow onion, shaved thin (see tip)
½ teaspoon black pepper
¾ teaspoon salt
3 small to medium red bliss potatoes, sliced ⅛ inch thick
8 large eggs, beaten, or 12 egg whites (for a lighter version)
1 tablespoon chopped Italian flat-leaf parsley, for garnish

WHAT TO DO

PREHEAT the oven to 325°F.

IN A 6-INCH SAUTÉ PAN, heat 1 tablespoon of the olive oil on medium heat. Add the onion and sauté for about 5 minutes, or until the onion is soft and has a little color. Season the onion with ¼ teaspoon salt and ¼ teaspoon black pepper. Set aside.

IN A 10-INCH nonstick, oven-safe pan, heat the remaining ¼ cup olive oil over medium heat. Fan the red potato slices in a circle, starting on the outside of the pan and working in, until the entire pan is covered, with very little of the pan showing through. A little overlap of the potatoes is okay, but not too much. Season the potatoes with ¼ teaspoon salt and the same amount of pepper.

COOK the potatoes on medium heat until they start to crisp, about 1 minute. Reduce the temperature to low and cook for another 5 to 7 minutes, until the potatoes are fork-tender. Spread the softened onion on top of the potatoes.

the
**BUSY
MOM'S
TIP**

A Japanese mandoline is great for slicing uniformly, but you have to be extremely careful with it. This tool is not meant for children. It's incredibly sharp and can easily slice your finger. It's better to use a slightly larger potato and throw away the last bit than to try to slice the last of it on the mandoline. Save your fingers. Throw away the last bit of potato.

WHISK ¼ teaspoon salt into the eggs and pour them over the onion and potatoes in the pan. Cook for about 30 seconds on medium heat. Move the pan to the oven and bake for 15 to 20 minutes. The frittata should look like an egg pie, and the center should be springy and firm to touch. If the egg is wet, it needs to cook a little longer.

SLIDE the frittata out of the pan and onto a plate. Slice it into 8 pieces, sprinkle with the chopped parsley, and serve.

THIS CAN ALSO BE SERVED at room temperature. If you want to refrigerate it to serve the next day, let it cool completely for 10 to 15 minutes and put it in the fridge, uncovered. Let the frittata cool for another 10 to 15 minutes and cover it with plastic wrap. Before serving, let it stand for an hour at room temperature, then warm it in a 475°F oven for about 3 minutes.

Buttermilk Biscuits with Honey Butter

More people would make homemade biscuits if they knew how easy it really is. For the honey butter, any butter you like will work, but for a real treat, try an Irish butter, available in most supermarkets, or a French butter, which you can find at high-end stores.

FOR THE BISCUITS

2 cups all-purpose flour, plus more for dusting

2 tablespoons baking powder

3 tablespoons sugar

1 teaspoon salt

1 large egg

¾ cup buttermilk or heavy cream

1 stick (½ cup) cold unsalted butter, cubed

3 tablespoons heavy cream

FOR THE HONEY BUTTER

1 stick (½ cup) unsalted butter, softened

6 tablespoons honey

WHAT TO DO

FOR THE BISCUITS:

PREHEAT the oven to 350°F.

COMBINE the flour, baking powder, sugar, and salt in a large bowl.

IN A SEPARATE BOWL, whisk together the egg and buttermilk. I usually measure the buttermilk in a liquid measuring cup and add the egg to it. Why dirty another bowl?

PINCH the cold butter into the dry ingredient mixture with your fingers until it becomes crumbly and all the butter is in small pieces. (You can also use a pastry cutter or a pair of spoons for this job, but I prefer to get my hands in the dough.)

If you don't have the right size cookie cutter, you can use a plastic cup to cut the dough into circular biscuits. One of my culinary instructors always said that fancy tools weren't necessary. He used an empty wine bottle as his rolling pin.

ADD your blended liquid ingredients and fold the mixture with your hands to form the biscuit dough. Knead the dough in the bowl for about 3 minutes. You don't want to overdo it.

LIGHTLY DUST a rolling pin with flour. On a lightly floured surface, roll out the dough until it's about 1 inch thick. You can cut it into circles with a pastry cutter or use a knife to cut it into squares to make 12 biscuits (see tip). Brush the tops with the 3 tablespoons heavy cream.

BAKE the biscuits on a baking sheet for 12 to 14 minutes. The tops and bottoms should be golden brown and firm to the touch. (If you have a convection oven, this is a good time to use it. The convection helps the dough rise and makes for a better biscuit. Baking will take only 8 to 10 minutes using a convection setting.)

FOR THE HONEY BUTTER:

WHISK the honey and butter together in a small bowl until they combine. Serve with the biscuits.

Cajun Country Potatoes and Sausages

The Cajun seasoning in this recipe is one of my favorites. It's a staple in my pantry. I also use it to make the Cajun Mayo (page 47) to go with my Aged Cheddar and Gruyère Mini-Burgers (page 47).

2 large russet potatoes, peeled and cubed

4 tablespoons canola oil

1 medium green bell pepper, cored, seeded, and diced

½ small red onion, diced

1 pound precooked smoked breakfast sausage, diced

2 tablespoons Cajun seasoning (your favorite brand)

WHAT TO DO

IN A LARGE BOWL, soak the cubed potatoes in warm water for 4 to 5 minutes to reduce their starchiness and prevent them from sticking in the pan. Drain the potatoes and rinse well under hot water. Pat them dry and separate them into two equal batches.

TO A 12-INCH SAUTÉ PAN over high heat, add 2 tablespoons of the canola oil and heat it until it starts to smoke very lightly. Add the first batch of potatoes to the sauté pan. Let one side cook for about 1 minute, without moving the potatoes around in the pan. You want to crisp the potatoes, and moving them around will prevent this.

ONCE THE POTATOES have browned well on one side, you should be able to shake them in the pan with little effort. Turn them over and let them cook for about 1 minute more, until the other side is brown.

TRANSFER the cooked potatoes to a bowl.

ADD the remaining oil to the pan, repeat the cooking process for the second batch, and then transfer them to the bowl.

ADD the bell pepper, onion, and sausage to the pan and cook it all for 3 to 4 minutes, until the vegetables soften and brown a little.

ADD the potatoes back to the pan, season with the Cajun seasoning, and stir well. Let it all cook for 2 minutes and serve.

Crab Cakes with Chipotle Adobo Aioli

MAKES 12 (2-ounce)
crab cakes

TOTAL TIME: 50 minutes

Like most college kids, I would come home looking forward to a home-cooked meal. After I started working at Spago, my parents were excited for me to come home and cook for them. Crab cakes were something I'd never had as a kid, but I perfected them in that first real job, and my family wanted me to make them whenever I visited. This brunch favorite always reminds me of the moment when the tables turned and I was the one doing the cooking for my parents.

the
BUSY
MOM'S
TIP

If jumbo lump crabmeat isn't in your budget at the moment, feel free to substitute crab claw meat or another less expensive alternative.

FOR THE CRAB CAKES

1 tablespoon unsalted butter

3 tablespoons finely chopped celery

3 tablespoons finely chopped shallots

2 tablespoons chopped cilantro, plus 1 tablespoon for garnish

1 (1-pound) can of jumbo lump crabmeat, picked over

1 large egg

1 tablespoon Old Bay seasoning

½ cup mayonnaise

1 cup panko bread crumbs, plus ¼ cup for shaping the cakes

1 cup vegetable oil

FOR THE CHIPOTLE ADOBO AIOLI

1 (4-ounce) can of chipotle peppers in adobo sauce

1 cup mayonnaise

WHAT TO DO

FOR THE CRAB CAKES:

OVER MEDIUM HEAT, melt the butter in a small sauté pan. Cook the celery and shallots in the butter just until they soften. You don't want to brown the veggies.

IN A LARGE BOWL, gently combine the cooked veggies, 2 tablespoons cilantro, crabmeat, egg, Old Bay, mayonnaise, and 1 cup panko. Incorporate the ingredients, but don't break up the crabmeat too much. Put the mixture in the fridge for about 10 minutes.

YOU CAN USE a 2-ounce ice cream scoop or ¼-cup measuring cup to measure equal portions for your cakes. To make them easier to form, dip the portion of crab in a bit of panko before shaping it. Shape the cakes into disks about an inch thick, not a flat patty.

PREHEAT the oven to 400°F.

STICK the crab cakes back in the fridge to chill for 15 minutes.

IN A LARGE SAUTÉ PAN, heat ⅓ cup of the oil on medium. Work in batches, adding ⅓ cup oil for each batch. Sear 4 crab cakes for about a minute on each side, until they're nicely browned. Transfer them to a baking sheet.

BAKE the crab cakes for 10 minutes. Remember, the crab and veggies are already cooked. At this point you're just cooking the egg and making sure the crab cake is warmed through.

FOR THE CHIPOTLE ADOBO AIOLI:
ADD the can of chipotle peppers and the mayonnaise to a blender and blend until the mixture is smooth and well incorporated.

SERVE the crab cakes on a platter. Garnish with the chopped cilantro, and serve the aioli on the side.

The Best Blueberry Muffins

MAKES 14 to 16 muffins
TOTAL TIME: 20 minutes

You can make these muffins with bananas, strawberries, or other fruit instead of the blueberries. Just dice the larger fruit into pieces about the size of blueberries. Bake these on a Sunday and grab them on the run on weekday mornings.

1½ cups all-purpose flour
½ cup sugar
2 teaspoons baking powder
⅓ cup canola or vegetable oil
1 cup buttermilk or whole milk
2 large eggs
1 cup fresh or frozen blueberries
Nonstick vegetable oil spray, for pan

WHAT TO DO

PREHEAT the oven to 325°F.

IN A LARGE BOWL, combine the flour, sugar, and baking powder.

IN A 2-CUP MEASURING CUP, combine the oil, buttermilk, and eggs. Pour the wet mixture over the dry ingredients and add the fruit while continually mixing with a fork. Don't use a whisk, which will just break up the fruit.

LINE the muffin pan(s) with cupcake liners, if you're using them. Spray the pan with nonstick spray. (Even if you use the liners, I recommend spraying the surface of the pan to prevent the muffin tops from sticking.)

USE a 2-ounce ice cream scoop or ¼-cup measuring cup to fill each muffin cup with an equal amount of batter.

BAKE for 12 to 15 minutes. The muffins should be golden brown and springy to touch.

Smoked Salmon with Crispy Potato Pancake

My mom is a quarter Jewish. Even though we're predominantly Italian, every once in a while I like to give a nod to the Jewish part of our heritage, and this dish is one way I do it. Regardless of your background, you can't go wrong with potato pancakes.

Juice of 1 lemon

1½ cups crème fraîche or sour cream

¼ teaspoon black pepper

3 tablespoons chopped chives

¼ cup capers

3 large russet potatoes, peeled and covered in cold water to prevent oxidation

Vegetable oil (up to 1 cup)

¾ teaspoon salt

1 pound presliced smoked salmon (see tip)

1 lemon, cut in half

1 small red onion, finely diced

WHAT TO DO

IN A SMALL BOWL, mix the lemon juice with the crème fraîche, black pepper, 1 tablespoon of the chives, and 1 tablespoon of the capers. Set aside.

USING THE LARGE HOLES of a cheese grater, shred the potatoes.

THE POTATO PANCAKES will need to be cooked in 3 equal batches. Add 3 tablespoons of oil to an 8-inch nonstick pan for each batch. Heat the pan over medium heat (see tip). Completely cover the bottom of the pan with the shredded potatoes about ½ inch deep. Pat the potatoes flat and season with ¼ teaspoon salt.

LET THE POTATOES COOK for 3 to 4 minutes without moving them around or scraping the bottom. You want a crispy crust to form and if you move the potatoes, you won't get that crust.

I prefer to use wild sockeye smoked salmon. Wild fish is like free-range chicken. It grows in its natural environment and has a better texture, a richer color, and more flavor than farm raised.

Stoves can vary greatly in temperature. Your medium might be my low; if you think you need to adjust the temperature, go ahead and do it.

28

USE a spatula to flip the pancake, adding more oil if needed, and cook for another 3 to 4 minutes, until the other side is crisp. Drain on a paper towel–covered plate. Repeat for each batch of shredded potatoes.

CUT the pancakes into quarters and arrange them on a platter. Add a healthy dollop of the crème fraîche mixture to the top of each one; about 1 tablespoon will do.

FOLD a slice of smoked salmon, almost like a rosette, and place it on top of each dollop of crème fraîche. You don't want to cover the entire pancake. It looks prettier if you can still see a bit of it.

SQUEEZE the 2 halves of lemon over all the salmon. Sprinkle with the onion, the remaining chives, and the remaining capers. Serve.

To seed the tomato,
simply quarter it and
run your fingers along
the inside, removing
the seeds.

Customized Mini-Frittatas

For Grandparents Day at my daughter's school, I make 570 frittatas using this recipe. It's not complicated and everyone loves the variety. *(see photo insert)*

Nonstick vegetable oil spray

12 large eggs

Salt to taste

Black pepper to taste

FOR 4 SPINACH-AND-FETA FRITTATAS

⅓ cup feta cheese

¼ cup shredded spinach

¼ cup chopped sun-dried tomatoes

FOR 4 TOMATO-BASIL FRITTATAS

8 basil leaves, torn

1 large tomato, cored, seeded, and roughly chopped (see tip)

1 tablespoon shredded or grated Parmigiano-Reggiano cheese (reserved)

FOR 4 CHICKEN SAUSAGE FRITTATAS

1 cup diced precooked chicken sausage

Mesclun greens or a fruit salad, for serving (optional)

WHAT TO DO

PREHEAT the oven to 350°F and spray a 12-cup muffin tin with nonstick vegetable oil spray.

BEAT the eggs in a large bowl and set them aside.

DIVIDE the ingredients for each type of frittata into 4 different tins, so you'll end up with 4 of each flavor.

DIVIDE the beaten eggs evenly among the tins. Season each one with salt and pepper and mix well.

BAKE for 15 to 17 minutes. The frittatas should rise and be springy to the touch. Pierce the center of one or two to test for doneness. If the egg is still wet, the frittatas need a little more time.

LET THE FRITTATAS COOL for about 4 minutes. Pop them out of the tin and arrange them on a platter. Serve with mesclun greens or a fruit salad, if you wish.

Cucumber-Watermelon Spritzer with Chamomile

the
BUSY
MOM'S
TIP

If you don't have a juicer, you can simply blend the cucumber and water-melon and strain the mixture through a strainer or some cheesecloth.

Most people think of iced black tea when they want a cold drink, but herbal teas, like the chamomile in this recipe, don't always have to be served hot. They make a great cold beverage, too. This drink is definitely more sophisticated than the average juice box, but I believe in introducing kids to a wide variety of flavors—and this recipe is easy to make. It's also great for adult guests at a brunch or other moms coming over for a play date.

1 large cucumber, peeled, seeded, and juiced (see tip, page 37)
2 cups watermelon, seeded and juiced (see tip)
24 ounces sparkling water
1 cup agave nectar
3 chamomile teabags

WHAT TO DO

COMBINE the cucumber juice, watermelon juice, sparkling water, and agave nectar in a large pitcher and blend well. Add the teabags to the pitcher and let them steep for at least 30 minutes. Serve over ice.

The Better Brown Bag

CHEESE AND CHARCUTERIE PLATE

SMOKED TURKEY AND GRUYÈRE PANINI WITH TARRAGON

BABY SPINACH SALAD WITH CHICKEN AND RICE

HOMEMADE HUMMUS

WHOLE WHEAT SPAGHETTI WITH BASIL PESTO

CHICKEN FAJITA TO GO

JASMINE BROWN RICE STIR-FRY

HONEY-YOGURT CHICKEN PITA POCKETS

CUCUMBER-AND-CORN TUNA SALAD ON BAGUETTE

I'M BIG ON GETTING KIDS EXCITED ABOUT THEIR LUNCHES. HOW MANY BROWN BAGS with a sandwich, chips, and an apple end up in the bottom of the cafeteria trash can? I'm not saying you should never pack that simple kind of lunch, but I think it's important to think beyond that. There shouldn't be much difference between what we feed our children and what we eat ourselves. Lunch is a great place to teach them the habit of eating real foods.

There are a few things I do to make school lunches more successful:

Invest in the proper containers and utensils. I found a reusable set that includes a fork, spoon, and chopsticks. A thermos is a must to keep cold things cold and warm things warm, and an insulated bag also comes in handy. Having their own lunch set to carry back and forth gives young children an opportunity to practice being responsible, too.

For dessert, throw a cookie in with a bag of dried fruit. That way, your child still gets to enjoy a treat but also starts thinking of fruit as a dessert option.

Give kids the chance to interact with the meal. With your help and supervision, kids as young as kindergartners can have a hand in packing their own lunch bag. And a simple thing like assembling a fajita at the cafeteria table helps children take ownership of their food, which makes it much more likely that they'll actually eat what you send with them.

When you're really in a rush and don't have time to put together lunch, head for the sushi section of your supermarket. Vegetable sushi (with no fish or seafood) and steamed edamame make better choices than most of the things marketed to kids.

Look for alternatives to the usual bag of chips. Baked chips are better than the usual deep-fried fare. Xea likes dried seaweed snacks and kale chips. There are new options on the shelves every day, and if you shop online, the choices are almost limitless.

The recipes in this chapter aren't just for the kids' school lunches. Double up—and make the same lunch for yourself, too. You'll save money, time, and calories.

Cheese and Charcuterie Plate

SERVES 2
TOTAL TIME: 7 minutes

Those prepackaged cheese, meat, and cracker lunches are incredibly popular with kids. Assembling your own is less expensive and puts you in charge of the quality of food your children (or you) have for lunch.

8 slices of salami (Xea loves sopressata)

8 slices of your favorite cheese (Xea loves Brie)

16 crackers (or a small baguette)

2 handfuls of grapes

2 handfuls of dried fruit (see tip)

2 handfuls of nuts (see tip)

1 tablespoon olive tapenade

WHAT TO DO

THIS RECIPE will make two separate lunches. Simply divide the ingredients to pack half of each in two reusable containers. Kids especially love to use bento boxes, which you can find online or at local retailers. The boxes are divided into separate compartments that keep foods from mixing, and the presentation makes the meal fun. Throw an ice pack in the lunch bag to keep the meat cool and the cheese from melting.

the
BUSY MOM'S TIP

Many school campuses are nut-free environments, since so many kids have nut allergies. Feel free to replace the nuts with seeds, or to not include either. In selecting the dried fruit, unsulfured, with no sugar added, is the healthiest option.

Smoked Turkey and Gruyère Panini with Tarragon

SERVES 2

TOTAL TIME: 10 minutes

You can always mix it up and substitute ham for the turkey, or use a different cheese. The goal here is to have a warm, toasty sandwich for lunch.

the BUSY MOM'S TIP

If you have a panini press, of course you can use it for this sandwich. Otherwise, the oven works just fine.

4 slices rye bread

1 tablespoon whole-grain mustard

4 slices smoked turkey breast

4 slices Gruyère or other Swiss cheese

¼ small red onion, thinly sliced

5 or 6 sprigs of fresh tarragon, chopped

1 tablespoon olive oil

WHAT TO DO

HEAT the oven to 450°F (see tip).

SPREAD each slice of bread with a quarter of the mustard, then assemble the sandwiches with the turkey, cheese, onion, and tarragon.

BRUSH the olive oil on a baking sheet and on the top of each sandwich. Don't worry about using all the oil.

PLACE a heavy ovenproof pan on top of the sandwiches to press them while they're baking. Bake for 6 to 8 minutes. Flip the sandwiches and press the pan down on them about halfway through the cooking time, just as you would press a grilled cheese sandwich with a spatula while it cooks.

TO KEEP THE SANDWICHES WARM, wrap them in parchment paper, then cover them completely in foil. They should still be warm for lunch.

Baby Spinach Salad with Chicken and Rice

I won a *Top Chef* Quickfire Challenge with a version of this recipe. It's a great use for leftover chicken, shrimp, or beef, and of course for leftover rice. Any kind of rice you have on hand will work, but my favorite for this recipe is Rice-A-Roni Chicken. If you need rice in a hurry, Uncle Ben's Ready Rice is done in 90 seconds, literally.

2 cups cooked rice (whatever kind you have at home)
½ cup cooked chicken
8 cherry tomatoes, halved
8 slices halved and seeded cucumber or hothouse cucumber (see tip)
1 cup baby spinach
8 kalamata olives, pitted
2 tablespoons olive oil
4 teaspoons sherry vinegar

WHAT TO DO

COMBINE the rice, chicken, tomatoes, cucumber, spinach, and olives in a bowl. Drizzle in the oil and vinegar and toss the salad well. Divide the salad between two reusable lunch containers. This dish can be served at room temperature, but I'd suggest an ice pack in the lunch box.

the
BUSY
MOM'S
TIP

I like to use hothouse cucumbers, because they have fewer seeds, but you can easily seed the conventional cucumbers you find in the super-market. Simply cut the cucumber in half lengthwise and use a spoon to scrape out the seeds.

Homemade Hummus

I like to pack this dip with a variety of crisp vegetables—carrots, celery, snap peas, peppers, cucumbers—along with pita chips, olives, and feta cheese.

1 (15.5-ounce) can of low-salt garbanzo beans (aka chickpeas)
¼ cup tahini (see tip)
3 tablespoons fresh lemon juice
½ garlic clove
Dash of salt
1 cup olive oil

WHAT TO DO

DRAIN the can of beans, reserving the liquid. Put the beans and half of the liquid in a food processor. Add the tahini, lemon juice, garlic, and salt. Process for 3 to 5 minutes, or until you get a smooth consistency.

STREAM the olive oil into the processor, just until it's blended in. The heat from the processor can make the olive oil taste bitter, so you want to have the oil in there for as little time as needed to get the job done. Stored in a covered bowl, this hummus will keep for up to 2 days in the refrigerator.

the
BUSY
MOM'S
TIP

Tahini is a ground sesame seed paste. I usually find it on the grocery aisle with "ethnic" foods— think Mediterranean, not Mexican—or with the canned foods. Occasionally, I find it in the refrigerator section near the guacamole.

Whole Wheat Spaghetti
with Basil Pesto

This is one of Xea's favorite dishes. When we eat out at Italian restaurants, she likes to order gnocchi with pesto, but gnocchi's a little labor-intensive to bust out for school lunches, so we make this instead.

1 cup fresh basil leaves

½ cup shredded Parmigiano-Reggiano cheese

½ cup olive oil

2 teaspoons salt

1 teaspoon black pepper

1 tablespoon pine nuts (optional, see tip)

*4 servings cooked, warm whole wheat pasta (cooked according to the
    package directions)*

WHAT TO DO

ADD the basil, Parmigiano-Reggiano, olive oil, salt, pepper, and pine nuts to a blender and blend on high for about 2 minutes.

IN A LARGE BOWL, toss the pesto and pasta together until they're well combined. Although this pasta tastes good at room temperature, I like to pack it in a thermos, so it's still warm at lunchtime.

the
**BUSY
MOM'S
TIP**

Leave out the pine nuts if this lunch is going to a nut-free school or work environment.

This sauce can be made the night before, but it takes so little time— you can cook it in the morning while you make breakfast.

Chicken Fajita To Go

This lunch is especially fun for kids, because they get to assemble the meal at school. A lunch they can interact with tends to be more appealing. Just double the recipe to make enough for yourself.

¼ cup vegetable oil

1 medium green bell pepper, cored, seeded, and sliced in ¼-inch strips

½ medium white onion, thinly sliced

1 chicken breast, halved and sliced in ¼-inch strips

2 teaspoons salt

Pinch of black pepper (about ¼ teaspoon)

1 tablespoon ground cumin

2 medium flour tortillas

Salsa, shredded cheese, shredded lettuce, and diced tomato, for garnish
(optional)

WHAT TO DO

IN A 10- TO 12-INCH SAUTÉ PAN, heat the oil on high. Add the bell pepper, onion, and chicken to the pan. Season the chicken and vegetables with the salt, pepper, and cumin, then sauté on high for 3 to 4 minutes, or until the chicken is cooked through.

PACK the cooked chicken, peppers, and onions in widemouthed thermoses to keep warm. The vegetables will continue to cook and soften a bit. Wrap the tortillas in foil. They will be fine at room temperature. Pack any garnishes in separate containers.

Jasmine Brown Rice Stir-Fry

The rice for this dish should be cooked the night before and stored uncovered in the fridge. Anytime you want to do fried rice, the rice needs time to dry out. Children tend to be more receptive to brown rice if they have it in a dish like this, rather than as a plain side dish. *(see photo insert)*

the
BUSY
MOM'S
TIP

When you are sautéing don't move the food around too much. Continually stirring it just creates moisture and prevents browning. Don't stir more than every 2 minutes.

2 tablespoons vegetable oil

1 chicken breast, halved and cut into 1-inch cubes

¼ teaspoon salt

¼ teaspoon black pepper

½ medium yellow onion, diced

½ medium red bell pepper, diced

½ cup chopped asparagus, or chopped broccoli florets

½ cup frozen edamame, defrosted

2 cups cooked jasmine brown rice

2 large eggs, lighty beaten

½ cup oyster sauce

½ cup chopped green onion

WHAT TO DO

IN A 10- TO 12-INCH SAUTÉ PAN, heat the oil on high. Add the chicken to the pan and season it with the salt and pepper. Sauté the chicken for 1 to 2 minutes, until there's no pink visible on the outside and it starts to lightly brown.

ADD the onion, bell pepper, asparagus, and edamame to the pan. Cook the vegetables for 4 to 5 minutes, tossing them every 2 minutes. You want the vegetables to get crispy and a little brown, so don't stir them too much (see tip).

ADD the rice to the pan, and sauté it all for another 4 minutes. While that cooks, scramble the eggs in a separate pan.

POUR the oyster sauce into the stir-fry and cook for another minute. Toss in the green onion and scrambled eggs.

Honey-Yogurt Chicken Pita Pockets

Yogurt makes a nice alternative to salad dressing, mayonnaise, or barbecue sauce, which can be high in sugar, fat, and preservatives. Honey yogurt is a healthier, lighter, more refreshing option.

1 whole pita

2 chicken cutlets or 4 to 6 chicken tender pieces

½ tablespoon olive oil

1 teaspoon salt

½ teaspoon black pepper

1 teaspoon Cajun seasoning (your favorite brand)

2 romaine lettuce leaves, roughly chopped

3 tablespoons canned corn

½ avocado, diced

1½ tablespoons chopped fresh cilantro

¼ cup low-fat plain yogurt

½ tablespoon honey

WHAT TO DO

HEAT the oven to 450°F.

SLICE the pita in half. If you have trouble getting the pockets to open, heat the pieces in the oven or in the toaster for a minute or two. They should open right up.

RUB the chicken with the oil and season it with the salt, pepper, and Cajun seasoning. Roast for 9 minutes, or until the center of the chicken is firm to touch.

WHILE THE CHICKEN COOKS, toss together the romaine, corn, avocado, and 1 tablespoon of the cilantro to make the salad.

COOL the chicken in the fridge for about 5 minutes.

IN A SMALL BOWL, mix the yogurt, honey, and ½ tablespoon cilantro.

COAT the cooked chilled chicken in the honey-yogurt mixture.

STUFF the chicken into the pita pockets and top them with equal portions of the salad.

Cucumber-and-Corn Tuna Salad on Baguette

Tuna salad is a lunch-bag classic. This recipe makes it a little more special by adding a few extra flavors and serving it open-face on a toasted baguette. (see photo insert)

1 (5- to 6-ounce) can of albacore tuna in water, drained

½ small cucumber, peeled and diced

3 tablespoons corn, canned or sliced raw from the cob (see tip, page 60)

1 medium tomato, cored, seeded, and diced (see tip, page 30)

1 tablespoon chopped Italian flat-leaf parsley

Juice of 2 limes

1 tablespoon mayonnaise

Salt to taste

Black pepper to taste

4 slices French baguette

1 tablespoon olive oil

2 hard-boiled large eggs, peeled and quartered

WHAT TO DO

PREHEAT the oven to 450°F.

IN A LARGE MIXING BOWL, combine the tuna, cucumber, corn, tomato, parsley, lime juice, and mayonnaise. Season with salt and pepper and mix well.

BRUSH both sides of the baguette slices with the olive oil and place them on a baking sheet. Bake for 2 to 3 minutes, just until warm.

DIVIDE the tuna salad into 4 equal parts and top each slice of bread with a portion. Garnish each slice with 2 quarters of boiled egg.

---

the
**BUSY
MOM'S
TIP**

If you're worried about transporting an open-face sandwich like this one in your lunch bag, don't be. Xea and I do it all the time. As long as you fit the sandwich into a container that leaves very little room for it to move around, it transports perfectly and even feels a little more elegant than the usual sandwich. You can also rest the sandwich on a few leaves of butter lettuce to make it fit the container more snugly. And the more kids see green leafy vegetables, the more likely they are to eat them.

School-Night Dinners

AGED CHEDDAR AND GRUYÈRE MINI-BURGERS WITH CAJUN MAYO

ITALIAN SAUSAGE HEROES WITH HORSERADISH CREAM SAUCE

SHRIMP-AND-SAUSAGE CORN CHOWDER

GRILLED FISH TACOS WITH CILANTRO CABBAGE

CROQUE MONSIEUR AND MADAME

PUREE OF TORTILLA SOUP

GRILLED SHRIMP WITH CHIMICHURRI

QUINOA-CORN SALAD

CHICKEN PAILLARD WITH BABY PEAS AND POTATOES

GRILLED CHEESE WITH TOMATO SOUP

FISH AND CHIPS WITH MALT VINEGAR AIOLI

SKIRT STEAK SANDWICHES WITH JALAPEÑO SAUCE

CHICKEN BOLOGNESE WITH RIGATONI

QUICK PASTA SAUCE

BAKED PENNE WITH THREE CHEESES

GRILLED SALMON WITH TOMATO, CUCUMBER, AND DILL RELISH

CHINESE CHICKEN SALAD

SHRIMP LO MEIN WITH BELL PEPPER, EDAMAME, AND SCALLIONS

HOMEWORK, SCIENCE FAIR PROJECTS AND BOOK REPORTS, SWIM PRACTICE, soccer practice, tennis practice, dance lessons and piano—I know how busy weeknights can be when everyone in the family has something going on. After a long day of school and work, it's tempting to just pull into the nearest drive-thru and get dinner in a greasy paper bag. We all do it sometimes. (Have I mentioned my love of french fries?) But we all know it's not the best food we can feed our families, and a quick meal in the car robs us of the opportunity to spend a few minutes of uninterrupted face-to-face time with each other.

To make home cooking a little easier on busy school nights:

- Keep your fridge and pantry stocked with the basics (see page 7).
- Plan the week's dinner menu in advance.
- Prep what you can the night before or in the morning.
- Use Sunday nights to cook double or triple batches of things like Tex-Mex Turkey Chili (see page 145) or the pasta sauce from Spaghetti and Meatballs (see page 159). Freeze the extra to serve on weeknights.
- Make cooking a family affair. Even small kids can set the table and help with cleanup.

The recipes in this chapter take thirty minutes or less to prepare, and if you recruit the kids to help you, some of the dishes can be done even faster. You may not have time for leisurely weekday dinners, but even fifteen minutes of engaging with one another over a good meal can make a real difference to your family, especially when you turn off the cell phones, the laptops, and the TV to focus on the food and one another.

Aged Cheddar and Gruyère Mini-Burgers with Cajun Mayo

MAKES 12 mini-burgers
TOTAL TIME: 20 minutes

I love butter lettuce with these burgers, but choose what your family likes. The same goes for the buns. I prefer the sweet rolls and kids love them, but any dinner roll will do. *(see photo insert)*

FOR THE MINI-BURGERS

1½ pounds 80/20 ground sirloin

2 tablespoons finely chopped Italian flat-leaf parsley

1 tablespoon chopped marjoram or oregano, or 1 teaspoon dried Italian seasoning (see tip)

¾ teaspoon kosher salt

¼ teaspoon black pepper

3 slices aged cheddar cheese, cut into quarters

3 slices Gruyère or other Swiss cheese, cut into quarters

2 tablespoons peanut oil (optional)

FOR THE CAJUN MAYO

1 teaspoon Cajun seasoning (your favorite brand)

½ cup mayonnaise

12 Hawaiian sweet rolls, sliced

Lettuce leaves, tomato slices, and onion slices, for garnish

the
BUSY
MOM'S
TIP

Dried Italian seasoning is a medley of marjoram, oregano, and parsley, so you can use it to replace any or all of those herbs.

You can substitute whatever your favorite cheese is. Mine is a really stinky blue.

WHAT TO DO

FOR THE MINI-BURGERS:

PREHEAT the grill to high.

IN A LARGE BOWL, combine the ground sirloin, parsley, marjoram, salt, and pepper just until the mixture is well blended. Shape it into 12 equal-size burger patties.

GRILL the burgers on high heat with the grill top open. For medium-done burgers, cook them for 2½ minutes on one side. Flip the burgers and grill for another

2½ minutes. Flip the burgers again and top each one with 1 piece of cheddar and 1 piece of Gruyère cheese.

(IF YOU DON'T HAVE A GRILL, the burgers can be cooked in a 10-inch nonstick pan. Heat the peanut oil on high. Cook the patties for 3 to 3½ minutes on each side for medium-done burgers.)

FOR THE CAJUN MAYONNAISE:

IN A SMALL BOWL, combine the Cajun seasoning and mayonnaise. Blend well, then brush the rolls with the mixture. Assemble the burgers on the rolls and top with lettuce, tomato, and onion.

Italian Sausage Heroes with Horseradish Cream Sauce

SERVES 4
TOTAL TIME: 30 minutes

I remember walking the streets of New York City as a child during festivals like the Feast of San Gennaro. Sausage and peppers was a standard dish at those events and at every weekend barbecue. Having these heroes for dinner is like having a little taste of those special occasions in the middle of the workweek.

FOR THE HORSERADISH CREAM SAUCE

¼ cup sour cream

1 tablespoon prepared horseradish or 1½ tablespoons horseradish cream

1 tablespoon whole-grain mustard

2 tablespoons honey

FOR THE HEROES

4 (6-inch) Italian sausages (any kind you like)

5 tablespoons olive oil

1 large green bell pepper, cored, seeded, and sliced in ¼-inch strips (see tip)

1 large yellow bell pepper, cored, seeded, and sliced in ¼-inch strips

1 large yellow onion, sliced ¼ inch thick

1 teaspoon salt

1 tablespoon dried Italian seasoning

1 (24-inch) loaf seeded Italian bread, cut into 6-inch pieces

WHAT TO DO

FOR THE HORSERADISH SAUCE:

COMBINE the sour cream, horseradish, mustard, and honey in a medium bowl. Whisk well and set aside.

PREHEAT the oven to 400°F.

the BUSY MOM'S TIP

When you're slicing a round vegetable, such as an onion or bell pepper, slice off one side and turn the vegetable over to rest on the side you've just cut away. That way, the vegetable rests on a stable surface. As you continue, rotate the vegetable so it's always resting on a flat side. This is a great lesson to teach kids when they're first learning to cut with a knife.

FOR THE HEROES:

LAY the sausages on a baking sheet and brush them with 1 tablespoon of the olive oil. Bake the sausages for 25 minutes, or until they're golden brown. About halfway through the cooking time, turn the sausages over so that both sides will brown.

IN A LARGE SAUTÉ PAN, heat 4 tablespoons olive oil on high heat until the oil starts to shimmer. The oil needs to be hot before you add the peppers and onion so that the cold veggies won't lower the cooking temperature too much. (The oil may smoke lightly, but if there's a lot of smoke, the oil has been destroyed, so you don't want to let it go that far.)

ADD the sliced peppers and onion to the oil. Season with the salt and cook for 5 to 6 minutes, stirring every 2 minutes.

REMOVE the pan from the heat. Add the Italian seasoning and mix well. Cover the pan with a lid and let it sit for 5 minutes. The trapped steam will finish cooking the peppers and onions. They should be soft.

PLACE 1 sausage on a piece of bread and coat it with the horseradish sauce. Top each sausage with some of the peppers and onion.

Shrimp-and-Sausage Corn Chowder

SERVES 4
TOTAL TIME: 35 minutes

Homemade soup always tastes better after it's had the chance to sit for a while. I like it best the second day, but you can make it in the morning and serve it for dinner, or start in the evening and have it on the table in half an hour. Either way, this chowder has a comforting creaminess without being overly heavy. *(see photo insert)*

¼ cup olive oil

1 pound ground sweet Italian sausage, without the casing

1 small green bell pepper, cored, seeded, and diced (see tip)

1 small red bell pepper, cored, seeded, and diced

1 small yellow onion, diced

2 teaspoons salt

2 tablespoons unsalted butter

⅔ cup all-purpose flour

1 cup whole milk

4 cups chicken stock, or equivalent Better Than Bouillon or bouillon cubes
    (see tip)

2 cups canned, frozen, or fresh corn

1 pound 16/20-count shrimp, peeled and deveined, fresh or frozen, chopped in
    thirds or halves (see tip, page 58)

2 teaspoons chopped fresh chives

WHAT TO DO

IN A 4-QUART SAUCEPOT, heat the oil on high. Add the sausage and break it up it in the pan. Cook the sausage, stirring occasionally, for about 5 minutes, until it's browned and crispy.

TOSS in the bell peppers and onion. Season with the salt and reduce the heat to medium. Sweat the veggies for 3 to 4 minutes, just until they soften. You want to retain the color and not brown them.

---

the
**BUSY
MOM'S
TIP**

When you're prepping ingredients for a soup, remember that, with the exception of noodles, everything should be chopped small enough to fit in a soup spoon.

If a recipe calls for stock and you have only bouillon cubes or Better Than Bouillon, use the following conversions: 1 cube bouillon plus 1 cup water equals 1 cup stock. 1 teaspoon Better Than Bouillon and 1 cup water equals 1 cup stock.

ADD the butter to the pan. After the butter is melted, stir in the flour. There should be enough liquid in the pan for the flour to be completely incorporated. Continue stirring for about 1 minute.

POUR in the milk and chicken stock, stir well, and bring to a simmer. Reduce the heat to medium-low and allow the chowder to thicken for about 4 minutes. Add the corn and taste to see if the chowder is well seasoned. If you find it lacks flavor, you may need to add more salt.

LET THE CHOWDER SIMMER for 15 to 20 minutes. Reduce the heat to low and add the shrimp. Simmer for 2 minutes (a little longer if the shrimp is frozen), until the shrimp turns pink and curls into itself. You don't want to overcook it.

REMOVE the chowder from the heat and let it sit for 2 minutes. Stir in the chives.

Grilled Fish Tacos with Cilantro Cabbage

MAKES 12 tacos
TOTAL TIME: 20 minutes

I like to use mahi mahi for my tacos. It's a durable fish that won't fall apart when you grill it. Swordfish is my second choice; cod will also work. For an extra kick, top these with Chipotle Adobo Aioli (page 25). *(see photo insert)*

FOR THE TACOS

1½ pounds mahi mahi, cut into 12 equal pieces

2 teaspoons salt

1 teaspoon black pepper

2 teaspoons ground cumin and 2 teaspoons ground coriander, mixed together

2 tablespoons vegetable oil

12 corn tortillas (see tip, page 100)

Chipotle Adobo Aioli (page 25)

FOR THE CILANTRO CABBAGE

1 avocado, diced large

¼ small red onion, diced

1 tablespoon chopped cilantro

Juice of 1 lime

⅓ cup shredded cabbage

1 teaspoon salt

the **BUSY MOM'S TIP**

If you don't have a grill, you can use a grill pan or broil the fish on high for 3 to 4 minutes on each side.

WHAT TO DO

PREHEAT the grill to medium-high (see tip).

SEASON both sides of the fish with salt, pepper, and the cumin-and-coriander mix. Lightly oil each piece and cook for 3 minutes on each side.

REMOVE the fish from the heat and let it rest for at least 2 minutes.

WHILE THE FISH IS ON THE GRILL, you can prepare the taco toppings. In a medium bowl, combine the avocado, onion, cilantro, lime juice, cabbage, and salt. Toss well.

TO WARM THE TORTILLAS, you can place them directly on the medium flame of a gas stove or heat them in a nonstick pan.

FILL each tortilla with 1 piece of fish, a teaspoon of Chipotle Adobo Aioli, (see page 25), and equal portions of the Cilantro Cabbage.

Croque Monsieur and Madame

MAKES 4 sandwiches
TOTAL TIME: 20 minutes

A croque monsieur is really a glorified grilled cheese sandwich with ham, but it's delicious enough to deserve that glory. A croque madame is the same sandwich with a sunny-side-up egg on top. Both are traditionally covered in cream sauce, but for a somewhat lighter option, I prefer to skip the sauce and serve them with whole-grain mustard on the side.

8 slices French bread such as brioche or pain de mie, or challah bread

8 teaspoons unsalted butter

12 thin slices Parisian ham (aka French ham), or your favorite roasted or boiled ham

2⅔ cups grated Gruyère or other Swiss cheese

4 large eggs (optional)

Nonstick vegetable oil spray (optional)

Whole-grain mustard (optional)

WHAT TO DO

PREHEAT the oven to 425°F.

SPREAD each slice of bread with 1 teaspoon butter. Assemble the sandwiches, buttered side out, with 3 slices of ham and ⅓ cup cheese on each sandwich. Put all the sandwiches on a baking sheet and pop them in the oven.

COOK the sandwiches for 6 minutes on the first side, or until the bottom is golden brown. Flip the sandwiches and cook for 4 minutes more.

TOP each sandwich with ⅓ cup cheese and return to the oven to cook for another 2 minutes, or until the cheese on top is golden brown and slightly crispy.

YOU CAN SERVE these as they are, or go from croque monsieur to croque madame by cooking the eggs sunny-side-up and laying one on top of each sandwich. (See cooking instructions for sunny-side-up eggs in the Open-Face BLT with Eggs on the Sunny Side recipe, page 15.)

I USUALLY SERVE these sandwiches with a side of whole-grain mustard and a nice salad.

Puree of Tortilla Soup

This soup is hearty enough to be served as a meal and makes a great vegetarian option. By pan-roasting or grilling the vegetables, you bring out a rich, complex flavor that really elevates the taste of the soup. It's worth the small extra effort.

2 red bell peppers, cored, seeded, and halved (see tip, page 49)

4 large tomatoes

1 medium yellow onion, sliced in half

1 jalapeño pepper (see tip)

6 tablespoons vegetable oil

1 tablespoon salt

¼ tablespoon black pepper

4 garlic cloves

2 tablespoons ground cumin

6 fresh cilantro stems, leaves reserved for garnish

3 cups vegetable stock, or equivalent Better Than Bouillon or bouillon cube
(see tip, page 51)

4 cups tortilla chips

Lime slices, sour cream, Mexican crema, and shredded cheese, such as cheddar,
Monterey Jack, cotija, or queso fresco, for garnish (optional)

If you don't have a grill, you can sauté the vegetables on high heat. Put the oil in the pan and add the vegetables. Stir them continuously for 4 or 5 minutes, until the vegetables take on some color.

All the heat of the jalapeño pepper comes from the seeds. Use more of them for more spice or leave them out altogether for a milder flavor.

WHAT TO DO

HEAT the grill on high (see tip). Throw the red peppers, tomatoes, onion, and jalapeño in a bowl and douse them with the vegetable oil. Season them with salt and pepper and lay them on the hot grill for about 5 minutes. Rotate them to get color on both sides. You want to get a nice char on the vegetables, which should be black in spots.

ONCE THE VEGETABLES ARE CHARRED, move them to a 6-quart saucepot and add the garlic. On medium heat, cook the vegetables for another 4 to 5 minutes so they can soften. Add the cumin and the cilantro stems and let them cook for 1 minute.

ADD the stock and the tortilla chips.

REDUCE THE HEAT to medium-low and let the soup simmer for 30 to 40 minutes. Taste the broth to make sure it's seasoned well. If it tastes a little bland, you probably need to add more salt.

WORKING IN BATCHES that don't fill the blender more than halfway, blend the soup until it's smooth (see tip). You can't blend this soup too much.

POUR the soup into a serving dish and serve with your favorite garnishes. I like fresh lime slices, the cilantro leaves, sour cream, Mexican crema, and a shredded cheese.

the
BUSY
MOM'S
TIP

When you're blending hot liquids, work in batches. Never fill the blender more than halfway. Take the stopper off the blender top and just cover that hole with dish towel. Pulse the liquid a few times to let some of the heat escape before you blend; otherwise the expanding heat can send the blender lid flying off and hot liquid spraying all over the place. This is not a time for kids to be in the kitchen.

Grilled Shrimp with Chimichurri

Shrimp is actually one of the easiest types of seafood to work with from a frozen state. You can just run it under cold water to defrost and pat it dry with paper towels. The important thing is to buy it already peeled and deveined. It makes cooking a lot easier.

■

If you don't have a grill, you can use a grill pan or cook the shrimp under a broiler set to high for 2 to 3 minutes on each side.

Chimichurri is an Argentinean flavored sauce. It's light, refreshing, and herbaceous—like a pesto, but without the cheese. The raw olive oil adds a nice flavor and since it isn't cooked, it retains all of its natural health benefits. Plus, chimichurri is quick and easy to make.

FOR THE CHIMICHURRI

1 bunch Italian flat-leaf parsley

1 cup olive oil

2 tablespoons fresh lemon juice

Grated zest of 1 lemon

1 teaspoon chopped fresh rosemary or ½ teaspoon dried rosemary

1 teaspoon chopped fresh marjoram or ½ teaspoon dried marjoram

1 garlic clove

¼ teaspoon salt

FOR THE SHRIMP

1 pound 16/20-count shrimp, peeled and deveined, tail on, fresh or frozen
    (see tip)

1 tablespoon salt

1 teaspoon black pepper

¼ cup olive oil

WHAT TO DO

PREHEAT the grill to high (see tip).

FOR THE CHIMICHURRI:

COMBINE the parsley, oil, lemon juice, zest, rosemary, marjoram, garlic, and salt in the blender. Blend on high for about a minute and set it aside.

FOR THE SHRIMP:

LAY out the shrimp on a large plate or baking sheet and season them with the salt and pepper. Massage them with the olive oil to coat evenly.

GRILL the shrimp for 2 minutes on each side, until they tighten and change from gray to a pinkish color.

ARRANGE the grilled shrimp on a platter and top with the chimichurri. Serve with a salad, vegetables, and rice, or Quinoa-Corn Salad (page 60).

Quinoa-Corn Salad

This salad is great to serve as a summer side dish, when fresh corn is in season. Frozen or canned corn is certainly okay to use when fresh isn't available, but when you can, use fresh corn on the cob. You'll taste the difference.

2 cups cooked quinoa (prepared according to package directions)

1 cup raw, fresh corn kernels (about 4 or 5 ears; see tip)

2 small radishes, shaved thinly (see tip, page 19)

2 tablespoons olive oil

1 tablespoon sherry vinegar, champagne vinegar, or white wine vinegar

WHAT TO DO

IN A LARGE BOWL, combine the quinoa, corn, radishes, olive oil, and vinegar and toss it all together.

THIS SIDE DISH is delicious with the Grilled Shrimp with Chimichurri (page 58) because the chimichurri sauce goes perfectly with the quinoa and corn.

---

the BUSY MOM'S TIP

Many people overcook corn when they prepare it. The beauty of corn is that you don't have to cook it at all. It's delicious straight from the cob. Removing the kernels from the cob is easy. Cover your cutting board with a paper towel or clean dish towel to prevent the kernels from bouncing off. Trim off the end of the cob so that you can stand it straight and make it safer to work with. Stand the cob on the covered cutting board and use a knife to slice off the kernels from top to bottom. Use the paper towel or dish towel to transfer the kernels.

Chicken Paillard with
Baby Peas and Potatoes

SERVES 4
TOTAL TIME: 30 minutes

This dish might sound fancy, but it's really just chicken pounded very, very thin. As you're pounding it thinner and thinner, you're tenderizing the chicken. If you don't have a mallet, you can use the flat side of the blade of a large knife to do the pounding.

FOR THE POTATOES

2 Yukon Gold potatoes, peeled, diced ⅛ inch, and covered in water
    to prevent oxidation

2 teaspoons salt

½ teaspoon black pepper

¼ cup olive oil

FOR THE CHICKEN

2 large boneless, skinless chicken breasts, halved, or 4 chicken cutlets

⅓ cup vegetable oil

2 teaspoons salt

1 teaspoon black pepper

⅓ cup all-purpose flour

FOR THE PEAS

2 tablespoons unsalted butter

1 cup frozen peas (or use fresh peas if you can find them; see tip)

2 teaspoons salt

½ cup water

1 teaspoon chicken Better Than Bouillon or 1 bouillon cube

2 lemons, sliced in half

2 tablespoons chopped fresh basil, for garnish

the
**BUSY
MOM'S
TIP**

If fresh peas are in season, shucking them from the pod is a great activity for the kids.

WHAT TO DO

PREHEAT the oven to 475°F.

FOR THE POTATOES:

SEASON the potatoes with the salt and pepper and toss them in the olive oil. Lay them out on a baking sheet and roast them for 10 minutes, until they are cooked through and soft, tossing every 3 minutes to brown evenly. Then set them aside.

FOR THE CHICKEN:

COVER a cutting board with a sheet of plastic wrap and lay the chicken breasts on top of it. Cover the chicken with another sheet of plastic wrap; with a flat mallet or the flat side of a knife, pound each chicken breast until it's very thin.

IN A 12- TO 14-INCH SAUTÉ PAN, heat the oil on medium-high.

SEASON each breast with the salt and pepper, then dust with flour on both sides (see tip). Cook the chicken for 1½ to 2 minutes on each side. If you don't have a large enough pan for both pieces, reserve 2 tablespoons of the oil to cook the chicken in 2 batches. Move the chicken breasts to a 12-inch baking dish. At this point, they're not yet fully cooked.

FOR THE PEAS:

REDUCE the heat to medium, discard the oil from cooking the chicken, and add the unsalted butter to the sauté pan. Add the peas, salt, water, and Better Than Bouillon. Cook for 4 to 5 minutes, until the peas are warmed through and their skins soften.

SCATTER the potatoes over the chicken in the baking dish. Spoon the peas and their cooking liquid over the chicken and potatoes. Squeeze the juice of the lemons over the peas and place the baking dish in the oven. Finish cooking the chicken for 4 minutes, or until it's firm to the touch.

REMOVE the dish from the oven and garnish it with the fresh basil.

---

the
**BUSY
MOM'S
TIP**

To dust the chicken, dredge it in the flour and the smack it between your hands to knock off excess flour.

Grilled Cheese with Tomato Soup

SERVES 4
TOTAL TIME: 30 minutes

I made this grilled cheese sandwich for a feature in *Parents* magazine. Three kids under the age of seven joined me for the day. When I pulled out the raisin bread and started putting apples on the sandwiches, they all freaked out. They insisted they did not like raisins and they thought it was just weird to put apples on a sandwich. My good reputation for cooking with kids was going to be blown in one day! Fortunately, every one of the kids was at least willing to try this sandwich. And every one of them loved it.

FOR THE TOMATO SOUP

¼ cup olive oil

2 teaspoons chopped garlic

2 (28-ounce) cans of crushed tomatoes

¼ teaspoon salt

¼ teaspoon sugar

Black pepper, to taste

1 cup heavy cream

4 sprigs of fresh marjoram leaves, chopped

FOR THE GRILLED CHEESE SANDWICHES

4 tablespoons unsalted butter

8 slices cinnamon-raisin or hearty white bread

8 slices Havarti cheese

2 medium Fuji or Golden Delicious apples, thinly sliced

WHAT TO DO

FOR THE SOUP:

HEAT the olive oil in a medium saucepan over medium heat. Add the garlic to the olive oil; heat it just until you smell it and hear it starting to sizzle. Add the crushed tomatoes, salt, sugar, and pepper. Mix well and let simmer for 20 minutes (see tip).

the
**BUSY
MOM'S
TIP**

The soup needs time to simmer. In the meantime, make and grill your sandwiches. By the time the bread is golden and crunchy, the soup will be ready to serve.

ADDING COLD CREAM to a hot pot can ruin the whole dish, so warm the cream in a small pot until it's just under a boil. Pour the hot cream into the soup and add the marjoram. Stir well and remove the soup from the heat.

BLEND THE SOUP with a hand blender. If you don't have a hand blender, you can use your countertop blender, but work in batches and be careful! The hot soup will expand, so be sure the blender jar isn't more than half full. Remove the cap from the blender lid and cover the hole with a dish towel. This will allow some of the heat to escape (see tip, page 57). Blend the soup until smooth and return it to the saucepan to simmer.

FOR THE SANDWICHES:

HEAT a griddle or flat-surfaced pan on medium-low heat. Butter the outside of each slice of the bread with ½ tablespoon butter. Assemble the sandwiches, dividing the cheese and apple slices among them.

PLACE the sandwiches on the griddle and cook until golden brown on one side. Raisins have natural sugar, so the bread will brown more quickly than most, about 3 to 4 minutes on each side. Flip to cook on the other side. Once both sides are golden and crispy, serve with the tomato soup.

Fish and Chips with Malt Vinegar Aioli

SERVES 4
TOTAL TIME: 30 minutes

For this dish, I like to use a meatier fish. Cod and halibut are good choices. They hold on to their moisture and rich flavor through the cooking process. They're also more forgiving if they have to sit for a while before being served.

FOR THE FISH AND CHIPS

2 quarts vegetable oil, peanut oil, or canola oil

8 (3-ounce) pieces of fish (about a pound and a half)

2 cups low-fat buttermilk

2 large russet potatoes, skin on

2 cups all-purpose flour

3 tablespoons Old Bay seasoning

FOR THE AIOLI

1 cup mayonnaise

6 tablespoons malt vinegar

2 teaspoons chopped fresh chives

1 lemon, sliced into wedges, for garnish

WHAT TO DO

FOR THE FISH AND CHIPS:

HEAT the oil to 325°F, verifying the temperature with a candy thermometer.

IN A SHALLOW DISH, cover the fish with the buttermilk and set it aside.

SLICE the potatoes in 1/16-inch slices. A mandoline works great for this job, but please watch your fingers (see tip, page 19). Place the slices in a bowl and rinse them a couple of times in cold water to remove the excess starch. Otherwise, they'll brown faster than they cook.

A countertop deep fryer
would be perfect for
making this dish. If you
have one, use it! If not,
you can use a heavy
6-quart pot to fry the
chips and the fish. Just
follow a few safety
precautions. Never fill the
pot more than halfway
with oil, since the oil will
expand when it gets hot.
Keep pot handles turned
inward on the stove top,
and keep kids far away
from hot oil. When you
add food to the oil, don't
overcrowd the pot, and
always have a slotted
spoon or spatula on hand
to stir the food if the oil
starts to bubble up. That
will help the oil settle
faster. Last, if you have
a paper towel–covered
plate nearby, be sure
to keep it away from
the heat.

DRAIN the potato slices and drop them one at a time into the hot oil (see tip). Use a slotted spoon to move them around and make sure they're not sticking to one another. Cook the potatoes for 7 to 8 minutes, until the oil stops bubbling. (The bubbles are created by the water cooking out of the potatoes.)

REMOVE the crisp potatoes from the oil with a slotted spoon and place them on a paper towel–lined plate to drain.

YOU CAN USE THE SAME OIL from the chips to fry the fish. Increase the heat to 350°F, verifying the temperature with a candy thermometer.

DRAIN the buttermilk from the fish.

COMBINE the flour and the Old Bay seasoning. Roll each piece of fish in the seasoned flour. Cook 4 pieces of fish at a time until golden brown, or about 3 minutes per batch. Drain the fish on a paper towel–lined plate.

FOR THE AIOLI:

COMBINE the mayonnaise, vinegar, and chives in a small bowl.

SERVE the fish and chips with aioli and lemon wedges on the side.

Skirt Steak Sandwiches with Jalapeño Sauce

MAKES 8 sandwiches
TOTAL TIME: 25 minutes

The jalapeño pickling liquid and pickled jalapeños spice up the dressing for these sandwiches. If you want to make it less spicy, you can leave out the chopped peppers. If you don't want it spicy at all, you can replace the jalapeño pickling liquid with liquid from a jar of pickles or with white wine vinegar.

1 (1½-pound) skirt steak (or substitute 1-inch-thick rib eye or New York strip steak)

2 tablespoons olive oil

¼ teaspoon salt

¼ teaspoon black pepper

1 cup sour cream

¼ cup pickling liquid from a jar of pickled jalapeño peppers

1 tablespoon chopped pickled jalapeño peppers

¼ medium green cabbage, shredded

½ medium red onion, thinly sliced

1 avocado

2 medium tomatoes (see tip)

8 French rolls (4 to 6 inches long)

WHAT TO DO

PREHEAT the oven to 350°F.

HEAT the grill on medium. Rub the steak with the olive oil and season it on both sides with salt and pepper.

ONCE THE GRILL IS HOT, grill the steak for 6 to 7 minutes on each side (see tip). Remove the steak from the grill and let it rest for 10 minutes before slicing it. If you don't have a grill, you can use a grill pan on your stove top.

WHILE THE STEAK IS COOKING, combine the sour cream, pickling liquid, and chopped pickled jalapeño peppers in a small bowl.

the
BUSY
MOM'S
TIP

Vine-ripened, beefsteak, Roma—there are so many varieties of tomatoes available at your local market. I'd suggest you get to know your produce guys. They can educate you about which tomatoes are most flavorful, and if you're really nice, they might just take out a knife and let you sample one.

Even if you tend to like your steak more rare, skirt steak should always be cooked to medium. Otherwise the layers of fat will make it too tough.

IN ANOTHER BOWL, combine the shredded cabbage and sliced onion.

QUARTER THE AVOCADO and slice each quarter into 4 thinner slices. You'll have 2 slices for each sandwich.

CUT the tomatoes into 8 slices each.

SLICE the French rolls without cutting them all the way through. You want them to look like a Pac-Man mouth, still attached on one side. Warm the rolls in the oven.

CUTTING against the grain, slice the steak into ¼-inch-thick pieces.

SPREAD both sides of the rolls with the jalapeño sauce and fill each roll with the sliced steak, cabbage and onion, tomato slices, and avocado.

Chicken Bolognese with Rigatoni

SERVES 6
TOTAL TIME: 30 minutes

This dish calls for a mirepoix, a mixture of diced celery, carrot, and onion. Of course, you can chop these fresh, but I totally cheat and use the pre-chopped mixture from Trader Joe's. If your supermarket carries it and it fits your budget, go ahead and spend the money to save the time.

the
**BUSY
MOM'S
TIP**

1 pound ground chicken (white or dark meat, or a mixture of both)

½ cup peeled and diced carrot

½ cup diced celery

½ cup diced yellow onion (about ½ medium onion)

1 tablespoon salt

½ tablespoon black pepper

1 tablespoon dried Italian seasoning

1 (24-ounce) jar premade spaghetti sauce (see tip)

1 pound rigatoni pasta

1½ cups shredded or grated Parmigiano-Reggiano cheese

6 tablespoons ricotta cheese, optional (for homemade ricotta, see page 134)

Chopped fresh basil or Italian flat-leaf parsley, for garnish

Instead of using sauce from a jar, make a double batch of sauce when you prepare Grandma's Lasagna (page 153) or Spaghetti and Meatballs (page 159) and freeze the extra. You can turn the frozen sauce out of the container and right into the pan. You don't even have to bother defrosting.

WHAT TO DO

IN A LARGE, shallow saucepot over medium heat, brown the ground chicken. Add the carrot, celery, and onion and season with the salt and pepper. Continue cooking for 6 minutes, then add the Italian seasoning. Cook for another 1 to 2 minutes, until the vegetables soften and take on a little color.

ADD the sauce to the pot and cook for 5 minutes to allow the flavors to meld.

COOK the rigatoni according to the package instructions. Add the drained rigatoni to the sauce and cook for another 3 to 4 minutes on medium heat.

SERVE the rigatoni and sauce topped with Parmigiano-Reggiano and a sprinkle of basil or parsley. In our family, we've always eaten rigatoni with a scoop of ricotta on the side. If it sounds good to you, add a tablespoon of ricotta to each plate.

Quick Pasta Sauce

It would be great to enjoy a sauce that's simmered for hours every day of the week, but when you're short on time, grab a box of pasta from the pantry and make this quick sauce to go with it. Even the youngest kids can tear the basil leaves or sprinkle on the Parmesan and arugula in this recipe. Older children with a little more kitchen experience can cook this sauce by themselves. Cook a one-pound box of pasta, toss together a simple salad, and you've got a weeknight meal ready to go in less than twenty minutes.

1 (1 pound) box of pasta (cooked according to package directions)

¼ cup olive oil (see tip)

2 tablespoons roughly chopped fresh garlic (about 6 cloves)

4 cups halved cherry tomatoes (see tip)

1 tablespoon salt

2 teaspoons sugar

¼ cup extra-virgin olive oil (see tip)

10 large fresh basil leaves, torn

½ cup shredded Parmigiano-Reggiano cheese

1½ cups fresh arugula

WHAT TO DO

IN A 10-INCH SKILLET, heat the ¼ cup olive oil over medium heat. Add the garlic and let it cook just long enough to take on some color.

THROW IN the cherry tomatoes. They'll cool off the pan and prevent the garlic from burning. Turn the heat up to high and cook the tomatoes until they start to break down. Add the salt and sugar.

REMOVE the pan from the heat and add ¼ cup extra-virgin olive oil and the torn basil leaves to finish the sauce.

SPOON the sauce over the freshly cooked pasta of your choice and top with the Parmigiano-Reggiano and arugula.

the
BUSY
MOM'S
TIP

Any inexpensive olive oil will work for cooking. Once it's heated, it will lose much of its flavor and nutrients. I like to use a higher-quality, more flavorful oil to finish a dish like this sauce.

This recipe is great if you have tomatoes that are overripe and can't be used in a salad or sandwich.

Baked Penne with Three Cheeses

I don't believe in serving kids macaroni and cheese every day. It should be treated as an indulgence, because that's what it is. This is my version of the classic macaroni and cheese Xea's grandmother makes. Older kids can easily make this by themselves. Add a big green salad and they can have dinner ready before you get home from work!

1 pound penne rigate pasta

1 stick (½ cup) unsalted butter

¼ cup all-purpose flour

3 cups heavy cream

¼ teaspoon nutmeg

1 tablespoon Lawry's seasoned salt

1 teaspoon black pepper

½ pound shredded whole-milk mozzarella cheese

½ pound shredded cheddar cheese

½ cup shredded Parmigiano-Reggiano cheese

½ cup dried bread crumbs (preferably panko)

WHAT TO DO

PREHEAT the oven to 350°F.

PREPARE the penne rigate according to the package directions, minus 1 or 2 minutes of cooking time (see tip). Drain, then pour the pasta into a 13- x 9-inch oven-safe glass pan.

IN A 4-QUART SAUCEPAN, melt the butter on medium-low heat. Whisk in the flour until it's dissolved. Add the cream to the pan. Add the nutmeg, seasoned salt, and black pepper and whisk the mixture until it's warmed through.

the
BUSY
MOM'S
TIP

When you're boiling pasta that you're preparing to bake (as in a ziti, lasagna, or macaroni and cheese dish), cook it a minute or two less than directed. It will finish cooking in the oven.

REDUCE the heat to low, and add the mozzarella, cheddar, and Parmigiano-Reggiano. Stir until you have a smooth cheese sauce.

POUR the sauce over the pasta and top with the bread crumbs.

BAKE for about 40 minutes, until the top turns a golden brown.

Grilled Salmon with Tomato, Cucumber, and Dill Relish

This is a fresh, light, healthy weeknight dinner that's great in summer, when tomatoes are in season. It pairs well with basmati rice and can be served room temperature, so you don't have to worry about keeping it warm.

FOR THE RELISH

2 vine-ripe tomatoes, cored, seeded, and diced into ⅛-inch cubes
(see tip, page 30)

½ cup diced cucumber (see tip, page 37)

½ small red onion, finely diced

2 tablespoons chopped fresh dill

2 tablespoons olive oil

Juice of 1 lemon

FOR THE SALMON

1½ pounds wild salmon, skin off, deboned, cut into 4 pieces

4 tablespoons olive oil

¼ teaspoon salt

¼ teaspoon black pepper

2 tablespoons extra-virgin olive oil, for serving (optional)

WHAT TO DO

TO PREPARE THE RELISH, combine the tomatoes, cucumber, onion, dill, olive oil, and lemon juice in a small bowl. Set it aside while you grill the salmon.

RUB each piece of salmon on both sides with 1 tablespoon olive oil and season it with salt and pepper.

ON MEDIUM-HIGH HEAT, cook the salmon for 2½ to 3 minutes on each side. Once it's cooked, arrange the salmon on a platter. If you like, you can drizzle a bit of extra-virgin olive oil on top (see tip, page 71). The health benefits of olive oil are lost in the cooking process, and this is a good chance to add flavor and nutrition to your dish. It's not a necessary step, but I like to do it.

SPOON the relish over the fish and serve.

the
BUSY
MOM'S
TIP

A candy thermometer that clips on to the edge of a pot or pan only costs a couple of bucks and makes deep-frying much simpler.

Chinese Chicken Salad

I was waiting tables at Chin Chin, a Chinese restaurant in Los Angeles, when I first tried one of these salads. I was blown away by the combination of crunchy, sweet, tangy, and spicy. It was completely different from what I grew up eating in my Italian-American family, and I loved it. That was the beginning of my love for branching out to explore other ethnic cuisines.

FOR THE DRESSING

1 cup unseasoned rice wine vinegar

1 tablespoon sesame oil

½ cup sugar

¼ cup peanut, canola, or vegetable oil

2 tablespoons toasted white sesame seeds

FOR THE SALAD

2 (8-ounce) rib-in, skin-on chicken breasts, halved

2 tablespoons olive oil

2 teaspoons salt

½ teaspoon black pepper

4 cups peanut, canola, or vegetable oil

¼ (12-ounce) package of square wonton wrappers, cut into ¼-inch strips

1 head of romaine lettuce, roughly chopped

1 head of Chinese cabbage, shredded

¼ medium red onion, thinly sliced

¼ cup chopped fresh cilantro

1½ tablespoons chopped pickled ginger

WHAT TO DO

FOR THE DRESSING:

PUT the rice wine vinegar, sesame oil, sugar, peanut oil, and sesame seeds in a jar. Shake well, until the sugar is dissolved. If you don't have a jar handy, just whisk the dressing ingredients in a medium bowl until the sugar is dissolved. Add the sesame seeds and stir well to blend the dressing.

FOR THE SALAD:

PREHEAT the oven to 475°F.

RUB each chicken breast with 1 tablespoon olive oil. Season each breast with salt and pepper. Place the breasts on a baking sheet and bake for 17 minutes, or until firm to touch.

WHILE THE CHICKEN BAKES, you can get started on the rest of the salad: In a 2-quart saucepot, heat the 4 cups peanut oil on medium-high to 325°F. Add the wonton strips and stir with a slotted spoon for 1 minute or until lightly browned. Remove the strips from the oil and drain on a paper towel–covered plate (see tip, page 66).

REMOVE the chicken from the oven and let it rest for 5 minutes. Remove the skin and bones and discard them. Shred the chicken.

IN A LARGE BOWL, combine the lettuce, cabbage, onion, cilantro, and pickled ginger. Add the shredded chicken and about three-quarters of the wonton strips. Pour the dressing over the salad and toss well.

GARNISH the salad with the rest of the wonton strips and serve. To put a fun twist on this meal, I like to use chopsticks and serve the salad in Chinese takeout boxes, which are sold at most party-supply stores. You can do the same with the Shrimp Lo Mein (page 78).

Shrimp Lo Mein with Bell Pepper, Edamame, and Scallions

Lo mein noodles are fun to eat and they make a great dish for kids to practice using chopsticks. *(see photo insert)*

1 (12-ounce) package of dried lo mein noodles (see tip)

1 teaspoon sesame oil

2 tablespoons peanut oil or vegetable oil

2 cups 16/20-count shrimp, peeled and deveined, tail on or off, as preferred
 (see tip, page 58)

¼ teaspoon salt

½ head of Napa cabbage, shredded

½ medium yellow onion, thinly sliced (see tip, page 49)

1½ cups frozen edamame, defrosted and shelled

1 red bell pepper, cored, seeded, and sliced thin

1½ cups oyster sauce

4 scallions, including whites, chopped

WHAT TO DO

COOK the lo mein noodles according to the package directions. They'll only take 2 minutes. Drain the noodles and rinse with cold water. Season with the sesame oil and set aside.

IN A WOK OR 14-INCH SAUTÉ PAN, heat the peanut oil on high. Add the shrimp and season it with a pinch of salt.

COOK the shrimp for about 1 minute, until almost done. They should be partially pink but still showing some gray and should still be somewhat flexible. Transfer the shrimp to a bowl.

ADD the cabbage, onion, edamame, and red bell pepper to the pan. Add ¼ teaspoon salt and sauté on high. As the vegetables develop color, keep stirring them until they're slightly browned.

REDUCE the heat to low. Add the shrimp and the oyster sauce and let it all warm through.

AFTER THE SAUCE IS WARM, add the noodles and remove the pan from the heat.

TOSS the noodles 3 or 4 times to coat.

GARNISH with scallions and serve.

Multi-Meals

ROASTED CHICKEN 101

CHICKEN AND DUMPLINGS

MADRAS CURRY CHICKEN WITH TURMERIC BASMATI RICE

CURRY CHICKEN SALAD WITH CRANBERRIES AND PINE NUTS

LEFTOVER CHICKEN LETTUCE CUPS

OVEN-ROASTED BROCCOLI

SICILIAN PASTA AND BROCCOLI

BROCCOLI AND SMOKED GOUDA SOUP

CORIANDER ROASTED CAULIFLOWER

CAULIFLOWER GRATIN

BRAISED BRISKET

BRAISED BRISKET TACOS

OLD-FASHIONED MEATLOAF

MEATLOAF PITAS WITH TABOULEH

PORK CHOP MILANESE WITH WATERCRESS
AND BLUE CHEESE SALAD

PORK CHOP SANDWICHES WITH HERBED MAYO

I DON'T UNDERSTAND PEOPLE WHO REFUSE TO EAT LEFTOVERS (ESPECIALLY SINCE SOME things, such as pasta sauce, soup, and chili, taste better on the second day). To me, leftovers are the perfect way to get the most for your money and your time. Some meals, like meatloaf and roasted chicken, will almost always leave you with extra when the meal is done. Rather than waste that food, or make yet another bread-meat-and-cheese sandwich, I like to find more creative uses for the surplus. That way, everyone feels like they're getting a whole new meal, something tasty and interesting rather than just more of the same.

Just like I recommend that you double or triple batches of pasta sauce and soup so you can freeze some for later, I also recommend that you cook more than you need of things like broccoli and brisket, so you can make recipes like broccoli soup and brisket tacos the next day with minimal effort. Every dish in this chapter connects to another dish, using your leftovers to create another delicious meal.

Roasted Chicken 101

In culinary school, I was taught that before a student moves on to complicated techniques, there are two things she needs to master: how to properly cook an egg and how to roast a chicken. Those skills are essential for every home cook to master, too. Roasting a whole bird might sound intimidating, but trust me, it's really a simple process, and you can save the leftovers to make Chicken and Dumplings (page 85) or Leftover Chicken Lettuce Cups (page 90).

1 (3½- to 4-pound) whole roasting chicken (see tip)

½ medium yellow onion, peeled

1 carrot, peeled and halved

1 stalk of celery, halved

4 sprigs of fresh thyme

¼ cup olive oil

2 tablespoons salt

1 tablespoon black pepper

WHAT TO DO

PREHEAT the oven to 475°F (see tip, page 91).

CLEAR the inside of the chicken, removing whatever you find in there, and pat the inside and outside dry with a paper towel. Stuff the onion, carrot, celery, and thyme inside the chicken.

RUB the olive oil all over the outside of the chicken. You want to massage it like it's had a hard day. The beauty of a roasted chicken is the crispy brown skin, and the oil will help you accomplish that.

SEASON the bird with the salt and pepper, drop it in a roasting pan, and let it sit for another 10 minutes to bring the temperature up just a bit more.

the
**BUSY
MOM'S
TIP**

Take the chicken out of the fridge about 10 minutes before you're ready to start prepping it for the oven. Letting it start to come up to room temperature will prevent the oven temperature from dropping when you put in the chicken to roast.

ROAST the chicken for 15 to 20 minutes per pound. A 4-pound chicken will take an hour to an hour and 20 minutes to cook. Starting off at a higher temperature will get a nice seal on the outside of the chicken, while making sure the inside cooks completely.

AT 40 MINUTES' COOKING TIME, reduce the heat to 400°F. Continue cooking for another 35 minutes.

THE BEST WAY to determine if the chicken is cooked is to use a meat thermometer. (They're inexpensive—I highly recommend purchasing one.) The thickest part of the chicken thigh should be 180°F. You never want to check the temperature of the breast. It's always the first part to be done. If you don't have a thermometer, puncture the thigh. If the juices run clear, the chicken should be done. If the juices are red, the chicken definitely needs more cooking time.

ONCE THE CHICKEN IS DONE, remove it from the oven. An hour, an hour and a half—you can't let it rest enough. The intense cooking process forces the juices and flavor to the center of the chicken. Resting time will allow them to redistribute evenly throughout the bird.

WHEN THE CHICKEN IS WELL RESTED, you want to take it apart so everyone gets the piece that makes them happy. Cut the breast into a total of 4 pieces, remove the wings, and slice off the thighs and drumsticks.

DRIZZLE the juices from the pan over the chicken pieces and serve.

Chicken and Dumplings

SERVES 4
TOTAL TIME: 25 minutes

When you make Roasted Chicken 101 (page 83), you can always roast two birds at the same time. That way, even if your family eats a whole chicken for dinner, you'll have extra for recipes like this one to get you through the week.

2 tablespoons unsalted butter

¾ cup diced celery

¾ cup peeled and diced carrots

1 cup diced yellow onion

1½ cups fresh or frozen peas (see tip)

2 teaspoons salt

½ tablespoon chopped garlic (about 2 cloves)

2 sprigs of fresh thyme

1 bay leaf

2 cups all-purpose flour

½ cup white wine

2 tablespoons chicken Better Than Bouillon or 6 bouillon cubes

2 cups rough-picked chicken

4¾ cups water

¼ cup heavy cream

WHAT TO DO

IN A 3- TO 4-QUART SAUCEPOT ON MEDIUM HEAT, melt the butter. Throw in the celery, carrots, onion, and peas. Season the vegetables with 1 teaspoon of the salt, and let them sweat on medium heat for about 3 minutes. You don't want to brown them, just soften them.

ADD the garlic, thyme, and bay leaf to the pot. Stir in 2 tablespoons of the flour and cook for another 2 minutes.

the
**BUSY
MOM'S
TIP**

If you don't have peas on hand, you can substitute green beans, chopped into pea-size pieces.

POUR in the white wine and bring it to a simmer. Let it simmer for 2 minutes.

ADD the Better Than Bouillon, the chicken, and 4 cups of water. Stir it well and add the heavy cream. Bring the soup up to a simmer. Let it simmer for 10 minutes.

WHILE THE SOUP COMES BACK TO A SIMMER, you should have time to make 16 dumplings. If you find it's taking you too long, just turn the soup down to a low heat until the dumplings are all ready.

IN A LARGE BOWL, add ¾ cup water and 1 teaspoon salt to the remaining flour. Using your fingertips, work the mixture together until it forms a dough. Knead it a bit to make sure all the ingredients are well blended.

DRY and flour your hands. Measure out 1 tablespoon of dumpling dough at a time and roll it in your hands to form a ball. As you form the balls, set them aside on a plate. Once all the dumplings are made, add them to the soup for the last 5 or 6 minutes of the soup's cooking time.

REMOVE the bay leaf and thyme sprigs before serving (see tip, page 88). Some people like to serve this dish over rice, but I find the chicken and dumplings provide enough substance to make this a satisfying meal on its own.

Madras Curry Chicken with
Turmeric Basmati Rice

SERVES 4 to 6
TOTAL TIME: 35 minutes

When I first met my mother-in-law, she would never let me cook. I had to earn the right to cook in her kitchen, and I knew she'd finally decided she liked me when she taught me how to make this dish. She was giving me the approval to cook for her son, so I guess I'd passed her test! Leftover chicken from this recipe is perfect for Curry Chicken Salad with Cranberries and Pine Nuts (page 89). *(see photo insert)*

FOR THE CHICKEN

4 chicken legs

4 chicken thighs

4 tablespoons madras curry powder

3 tablespoons salt

½ tablespoon black pepper

¼ cup vegetable oil

¾ cup diced celery

¾ cup peeled and diced carrot

1 cup diced yellow onion (about 1 medium onion)

2 sprigs of fresh thyme (see tip, page 88)

¼ cup all-purpose flour

2 medium russet potatoes, peeled and diced

1 medium tomato, diced

1½ tablespoons chicken Better Than Bouillon or about 4 bouillon cubes

4 cups water

1 bay leaf (see tip, page 88)

FOR THE RICE

2 tablespoons vegetable oil

½ medium yellow onion, diced

½ cup fresh or frozen peas

1 tablespoon salt

½ tablespoon turmeric

½ teaspoon ground coriander

2 cups basmati rice, rinsed and drained

1 tablespoon chicken Better Than Bouillon or 3 bouillon cubes

4 cups cold water

3 tablespoons chopped fresh cilantro

WHAT TO DO

FOR THE CHICKEN:

IN A LARGE BOWL, season your chicken with 2 tablespoons of the curry powder, 2 tablespoons of the salt, and the black pepper. Rub it into the chicken.

IN A 4-QUART SAUCEPOT, heat the vegetable oil on high. If you can't fit all the chicken in the bottom of the pot, just work in batches. Brown the chicken on all sides.

REMOVE the chicken from the pot and add the celery, carrot, and onion. Stir in 2 tablespoons curry powder, 1 tablespoon salt, the thyme, and the flour. Reduce the heat to medium and cook for 2 to 3 minutes, stirring once or twice. The goal here is to bloom the curry, enhancing its flavor, and to soften the vegetables.

RETURN the chicken to the pot and add the potatoes, tomato, Better Than Bouillon, water, and bay leaf. Bring the mixture back to a simmer, then simmer for 20 minutes. It should be like a stew with a thick broth.

FOR THE RICE:

HEAT the vegetable oil in a 2-quart saucepot. Add the onion and peas and let them sweat on medium heat for about 3 minutes. Add the salt, turmeric, and coriander. Cook for another 2 minutes.

STIR the rice into the pot, coating it with the mixture of vegetables and seasonings. Toast the rice for about 1 minute.

ADD Better Than Bouillon and water to the pot, stirring to make sure the bouillon breaks up. Cover the pot and cook on medium-low for 15 minutes.

TOP the cooked rice with chopped cilantro and serve with the curried chicken.

Curry Chicken Salad with Cranberries and Pine Nuts

SERVES 4
TOTAL TIME: 15 minutes

This dish is quick and easy, but has more flavor than the typical chicken salad. Although here it's served over greens, it's also great for sandwiches. The chicken salad is especially tasty with the leftovers from Madras Curry Chicken (page 87), but you can use any leftover chicken you have. *(see photo insert)*

4 tablespoons raw pine nuts

2 cups (1 pound) chopped cooked chicken, a mix of white and dark meat

1/3 cup mayonnaise

8 teaspoons chopped fresh cilantro

4 teaspoons chopped red onion

2 teaspoons curry powder

1/4 cup dried cranberries

Salt to taste

Black pepper to taste

8 cups mesclun greens

1 lime, halved

WHAT TO DO

HEAT a sauté pan on low. Add the pine nuts to the pan and let them toast, stirring occasionally, for 5 to 6 minutes, until golden brown.

IN A LARGE BOWL, mix the chicken, mayonnaise, cilantro, red onion, curry powder, cranberries, and toasted pine nuts. Season the mixture with salt and pepper and spoon the chicken salad over the mesclun greens. Squeeze the lime over the salad just before serving.

Leftover Chicken Lettuce Cups

Chicken nuggets, chicken tenders, roasted chicken—chicken seems to be the one thing we always bring home after a restaurant meal. Although this recipe came from trying to find a more interesting use for Xea's leftovers, you can also use the meat from any home-cooked chicken.

1½ cups chopped leftover chicken, with any bones removed

¼ cup chopped cucumber (see tip, page 37)

1 cup halved cherry tomatoes

¼ cup crumbled feta cheese

1 teaspoon dried Italian seasoning or 2 teaspoons fresh marjoram
    (see tip, page 47)

12 kalamata olives, pitted and chopped

1 tablespoon whole capers

1 tablespoon olive oil

2 teaspoons sherry vinegar or white wine vinegar

¼ teaspoon salt

¼ teaspoon black pepper

1 head of butter lettuce (also known as Boston lettuce; see tip)

WHAT TO DO

IN A LARGE BOWL, combine the chicken, cucumber, tomatoes, feta cheese, Italian seasoning, olives, capers, olive oil, vinegar, salt, and pepper. Fill the lettuce cups (see tip) with the mixture and serve.

Oven-Roasted Broccoli

SERVES 4 to 6
(with leftovers)
TOTAL TIME: 20 minutes

Some kids might cringe at the sight of broccoli on their plates. But that's just because so many people still think the best way to cook broccoli is to boil it to death. Not only does that leave most of the nutrients behind in the water, but you also end up with a soggy side dish that most kids (and adults) find unappealing. Roasting the broccoli at high heat will caramelize it and give it a rich, nutty flavor that kids and adults both love. Save the leftovers to make Sicilian Pasta and Broccoli (page 92) or Broccoli and Smoked Gouda Soup (page 94).

6 medium to large heads of broccoli
1¼ cups olive oil
2 teaspoons salt

WHAT TO DO

PREHEAT the oven to 450°F (see tip).

CHOP the broccoli into florets, reserving the stems to make Broccoli and Smoked Gouda Soup (page 94) later in the week.

PLACE THE FLORETS IN A LARGE BOWL. Drizzle them with the olive oil and toss well. It may seem like a lot of oil, but broccoli is porous and will easily absorb the oil.

SEASON the broccoli with salt and transfer it to a large baking sheet, leaving at least ½ inch of space between all the pieces. If the broccoli is too crowded on the baking sheet, it will steam instead of roasting. If your baking sheet isn't big enough, just roast the broccoli on two baking sheets, using both oven racks. Move the bottom sheet to the top rack halfway through the roasting process.

ROAST the broccoli until the edges are slightly brown, for about 10 to 12 minutes, without moving it around on the pan. The bottoms of each piece should be nicely browned.

the
BUSY MOM'S TIP

So many people are scared to turn their oven above 350°F. To roast anything, you need your oven really hot. At the lower temperature, you're just baking and you won't get the nutty-brown color you'll get with the roasting. Go ahead and turn the dial past 350°F.

Sicilian Pasta and Broccoli

This is a simple dish my grandmother made for me when I was a child. Now I make it for my daughter, Xea, and she loves it. As the broccoli takes on a toasty brown color, it develops a delicious nutty flavor that even picky kids will like. You can make this with fresh broccoli or with the leftovers from Oven-Roasted Broccoli (page 91).

I recommend sautéing the broccoli in a shallow sauté pot, rather than in a sauté pan. You'll be able to sauté the vegetables properly and the pot will be big enough to accommodate the pasta after it and the broccoli are both cooked. If you don't have a sauté pot, use a sauté pan for the broccoli and combine the cooked pasta and broccoli in a large bowl.

1 cup olive oil, or more if needed (or ½ cup if using leftover roasted broccoli; see page 91)

2 large heads broccoli, cut in 1-inch florets (about 6 cups)

1 tablespoon salt (if using fresh broccoli)

8 garlic cloves, roughly chopped

1 pound penne rigate (Penne rigate is my favorite because the ridges give it more texture.)

½ cup shredded or grated Parmigiano-Reggiano cheese

2 tablespoons chopped Italian flat-leaf parsley, for garnish

WHAT TO DO

HEAT the water for your pasta while you prepare the broccoli.

FOR LEFTOVER BROCCOLI THAT'S ALREADY COOKED:

HEAT the ½ cup oil over medium heat in a shallow, 10-inch sauté pot (see tip). Cook the garlic only until it starts to lightly brown. Toss in the cooked broccoli and let it cook for about 2 minutes, just to warm it through. Take the broccoli off the heat and set it aside.

FOR FRESH BROCCOLI:

IN A SHALLOW, 10-inch sauté pot, heat the 1 cup olive oil over medium-high heat (see tip). Add the broccoli to the oil and season it with salt. Sauté the broccoli for about 4 minutes, or until it takes on a toasty color. The broccoli will absorb a lot of the oil, so if you find your pan getting dry, just add a little more oil to it. Throw in the garlic and cook for about another minute, until it's slightly brown. Don't burn the garlic! Take the broccoli off the heat and set it aside.

PREPARE the penne according to the package directions. Drain the pasta and toss it in the pot with the broccoli, garlic, and olive oil. If the mixture seems dry, add a little more oil.

TOSS in the Parmigiano-Reggiano cheese, stir, and garnish with parsley.

Broccoli and Smoked Gouda Soup

If you want to cut back on the calories and fat in this dish, you can substitute whole milk for the heavy cream. And if you can't find Gouda, feel free to top the soup with cheddar.

If you have leftover steamed broccoli, Oven-Roasted Broccoli (page 91), or broccoli from a recipe like Sicilian Pasta and Broccoli (page 92), this soup is a great place to use it. You can combine raw and cooked pieces, and don't throw away those stems. Just peel them and use them in the soup, or skip the peeling and strain the blended soup through a fine strainer. This recipe also works great with leftover cauliflower.

½ stick (¼ cup) unsalted butter

1 medium yellow onion, roughly chopped (see tip, page 49)

¼ teaspoon salt

4 cups roughly chopped broccoli florets and stems

2 cups water

2 cups heavy cream (see tip)

1 teaspoon liquid smoke, applewood or your favorite flavor

1 tablespoon (vegetable or chicken flavor) Better Than Bouillon or
   3 bouillon cubes

1 cup fresh spinach (optional)

1 cup grated smoked Gouda (see tip)

WHAT TO DO

IN A 4-QUART SAUCEPAN, heat the butter over medium heat. Add the onion to the pan and allow it to slowly sweat for about 5 minutes, until it becomes warm and translucent. You don't want to get any color on it. Season it with ¼ teaspoon salt.

ADD the broccoli to the pan and let it cook with the onion for another 5 to 6 minutes. The vegetables will sweat out their own liquid, which releases a beautiful flavor into the soup.

COVER the vegetables with the water and cream and add the liquid smoke and Better Than Bouillon. Let it all simmer on low heat for about 30 minutes.

TAKE the stopper out of the blender lid and cover the hole with a dish cloth to allow some of the heat to escape. Working in batches, so the blender is never filled more than halfway, add the soup to the blender, and pulse a few times to release some of the heat (see tip, page 57). Blend the soup until it's smooth.

IF YOU WANT THE SOUP to have a nice green color, blend in the fresh spinach.

POUR the soup into a serving dish and top it with the Gouda cheese. Serve it with some of your favorite garnishes, such as chopped green onions or scallions, or even some leftover kale chips from A Duo of Chips (page 114).

Coriander Roasted Cauliflower

Since you're already cooking, you might as well make enough to get a jump start on tomorrow's dinner. This recipe makes enough to serve as a side dish for four people and have leftovers for the Cauliflower Gratin (page 97) or the Broccoli and Smoked Gouda Soup (page 94) with cauliflower subbed for broccoli. If you're planning to make the soup, don't forget to save the cauliflower stems. This side dish can be served with Roasted Chicken 101 (page 83).

2 heads of cauliflower

1 cup olive oil

2½ teaspoons ground coriander

3 tablespoons salt

1 tablespoon black pepper

WHAT TO DO

PREHEAT the oven to 450°F (see tip, page 91).

SEPARATE the cauliflower florets from the stems and discard the leaves. Cut the florets into 2-inch pieces. In a large bowl, cover the florets with the olive oil. Season them with the coriander, salt, and black pepper. Toss it all very well to make sure the cauliflower is coated.

SPREAD the florets over two baking sheets. Make sure the cauliflower isn't crowded. There should be space between the florets. If not, they'll steam instead of roast and won't get the caramelization you're going for.

ROAST the cauliflower for 17 to 20 minutes, stirring the florets every 7 minutes. If you're using two racks in the oven, rotate the baking sheets each time you stir the cauliflower.

WHEN IT'S DONE, this dish should have a beautiful golden brown color.

Cauliflower Gratin

SERVES 4

TOTAL TIME: 45 minutes

Years ago, I worked as the banquet chef for Spago, Wolfgang Puck's restaurant in Beverly Hills, where I was serving parties of more than a hundred people. I made huge vats of potato gratin and obsessively perfected the technique for that dish. Eventually, I wanted to do something different, and cauliflower had the perfect texture to replace the potatoes. This gratin goes great with almost any meat as a main course, including the Braised Brisket (page 98). Leftovers from Coriander Roasted Cauliflower (page 96) can be used to make this dish.

4 cups cooked cauliflower florets (see tip)

½ cup grated Parmigiano-Reggiano cheese

2 cups heavy cream

1 garlic clove, smashed

1 sprig of fresh thyme

1 teaspoon salt

2 tablespoons panko or Italian-seasoned bread crumbs

WHAT TO DO

PREHEAT the oven to 350°F.

IN AN 8 X 8-INCH BAKING DISH, toss the florets with the Parmesan cheese.

IN A SAUCEPOT, heat the cream, garlic, thyme, and salt over medium heat. Once it simmers, remove the pot from the heat and allow the cream to steep for 10 minutes to infuse it with all the flavors.

REMOVE the garlic and thyme from the cream, then pour the cream over the cauliflower. Top with panko.

BAKE the gratin for 30 minutes, or until it's golden and bubbly. Let it sit for a few minutes before serving so the whole thing will be thicker and creamier.

the **BUSY MOM'S TIP**

Broccoli and cauliflower are often interchangeable, and this is another case where that's true. If you have leftover broccoli, you can substitute it for the cauliflower in this recipe.

SERVES 4 (with leftovers)
PREP TIME: 30 minutes
COOKING TIME: 2 to 3 hours

Braised Brisket

This is one of those dishes my grandmother used to make all the time. She'd stand over me and insist the only thing you needed to cook brisket was catsup and onions. These days, I like to use a little more than that, but like my grandmother, I always braise the brisket. Braised meats are great to serve as an entrée, but I also like to serve the leftovers over pasta or use them to make Braised Brisket Tacos (page 100).

1 (3-pound) brisket

¼ cup salt

1 tablespoon black pepper

¼ cup vegetable oil

1 carrot, peeled and roughly chopped

1 medium yellow onion, roughly chopped (see tip, page 49)

2 stalks of celery, roughly chopped

4 cups dry red wine

1 tablespoon beef Better Than Bouillon or 3 bouillon cubes

2 tablespoons tomato paste

*6 sprigs of fresh herbs (any combination of 2 sprigs each of rosemary, thyme,
    parsley, or oregano; see tip)*

WHAT TO DO

THE BRISKET can be braised in a Crock-Pot or a pressure cooker, or on the stove top or in the oven—whichever works best for you. If you choose to use the oven, preheat it to 375°F.

IF YOU HAVE a roasting pan that's big enough to fit the shape of the brisket, you can use that to sear the brisket on your stove top. If not, use a 6-quart saucepot and cut the brisket in half to fit.

the
BUSY
MOM'S
TIP

I'm not too picky about which herbs you use in this dish. If you have only one herb, then use that. I like to buy the poultry mixes, made up of three or four different herbs, from the grocery store. I just pick out the herbs I want to use. That way, I get a variety of herbs without having to buy whole bunches of each one.

SEASON the brisket with the salt and pepper.

HEAT THE OIL in the saucepot or roasting pan on high. Cook the brisket for about 5 minutes on each side to sear it well. Remove the meat from the pan and add the carrot, onion, and celery to the pan. Roast the vegetables for about 5 minutes until they start to brown.

SHIMMY the meat back into the pan, or if you're using the Crock-Pot, pressure cooker, or a different pan, move the meat and vegetables there.

ADD the red wine. Anything you have around the house is fine. (Well, anything but Manischewitz. Even my Jewish grandmother would say that's too sweet.) Cover the brisket with water and add the Better Than Bouillon, tomato paste, and fresh herbs.

COOKING OPTIONS

OVEN: 3 hours at 375°F
SAUCEPOT: 3 hours on low, with the pot tightly covered with a lid or foil
CROCK-POT: 3 hours on low
PRESSURE COOKER: 2 hours on medium-low

ONCE THE BRISKET is done cooking, remove the pot or pan from the heat, and let the meat rest for 30 minutes in the juices. Use a spoon to skim any fat off the top of the liquid.

IF THE SAUCE isn't thick enough, transfer it to a medium saucepot and cook it over medium heat until it reduces to the thickness you want. Then return it to the cooking vessel.

SLICE the brisket and put it back in the sauce.

I LIKE TO SERVE brisket with mashed potatoes or Cauliflower Gratin (page 97).

Braised Brisket Tacos

You don't need any dairy, like sour cream or cheese, for these tacos. The combination of the richness of the brisket and the freshness of the veggies is delicious on its own, and your leftover Braised Brisket (page 98) will taste like a whole new meal.

1 to 2 cups picked brisket, with cooking liquid

1½ cups shredded cabbage or shredded romaine lettuce

¼ cup shaved red onion (see tip, page 19)

2 small radishes, shaved

2 tablespoons chopped fresh cilantro

Juice of 2 limes

8 corn tortillas (see tip)

1 avocado, sliced

WHAT TO DO

IN A SMALL PAN, warm the brisket with the leftover cooking liquid.

IN A MEDIUM BOWL, combine the cabbage, onion, radishes, cilantro, and lime juice.

WARM the tortillas over a medium flame or in a pan on medium heat.

ASSEMBLE the tacos with the meat and veggies and top with the avocado slices.

the
BUSY
MOM'S
TIP

Corn tortillas, like the ones used here, have greater nutritional value than flour tortillas.

Old-Fashioned Meatloaf

SERVES 4 (with leftovers)
TOTAL TIME: 60 minutes

Using ground beef alone makes meatloaf taste fattier than I like, so I combine it with ground turkey. Don't worry. This takes only about 10 minutes to prep. The rest of the time, the meatloaf is in the oven doing its own thing. This recipe will give you enough servings to make Meatloaf Pitas with Tabouleh (page 103) for the next day's lunch.

1½ pounds 85/15 ground beef

1½ pounds ground turkey (dark or white meat, or a mixture of both)

2 tablespoons salt

1 teaspoon black pepper

2 tablespoons chopped fresh dill

2 large eggs

1 tablespoon Worcestershire sauce

1 carrot, finely diced (see tip)

1 stalk of celery, finely diced

1 medium yellow onion, finely diced

1 cup catsup

the
**BUSY
MOM'S
TIP**

If you don't want to spend the time dicing the carrot, celery, and onion, you can roughly chop them and then pulse them in a mini food processor until they reach a fine dice.

WHAT TO DO

PREHEAT the oven to 400°F.

IN A LARGE BOWL, combine the beef, turkey, salt, pepper, dill, eggs, Worcestershire sauce, carrot, celery, and onion. Mix it all just until it's incorporated. If you mix it too much, your meatloaf will be too tough.

A LARGE POUND CAKE PAN is perfect for making meatloaf. Spread the meat mixture evenly in the pan and pour the catsup over it. Cover the pan with aluminum foil and bake it for about 40 minutes, or until the meatloaf comes away from the sides of the pan and is firm to touch.

REMOVE the foil. (If the top of the meatloaf has too much liquid or fat on it for your liking, add enough catsup to cover it.) Cook for another 10 minutes, until the catsup forms a nice coating on top of the meatloaf.

LET IT REST FOR 15 MINUTES before draining the excess liquid. Shimmy the meatloaf out of the pan and onto a platter. I like to serve it with Shallot-Potato Gratin (page 171) or Rosemary Mashed Potatoes (page 158).

Meatloaf Pitas with Tabouleh

A dinner of Old-Fashioned Meatloaf (page 101) means leftover meatloaf for the next day. The usual meatloaf sandwiches are always delicious, but don't you sometimes want something different? Inspired by kibbeh, a ground lamb dish, this recipe lends a Middle Eastern flair to your leftovers and stretches them further, too.

3 Roma tomatoes, cored, seeded, and diced (see tips, pages 30 and 67)

1 cup bulgur wheat, cooked according to package directions

6 large sprigs of fresh mint, torn

2 tablespoons chopped green onion

¼ cup chopped curly parsley

2 tablespoons fresh lemon juice

⅓ cup diced cucumber (see tip, page 37)

⅓ cup crumbled feta

2 cups diced leftover meatloaf

4 pita rounds, cut in half

WHAT TO DO

IN A LARGE BOWL, combine the tomatoes, bulgur wheat, mint, green onion, parsley, lemon juice, cucumber, feta, and meatloaf—everything but the pitas. Stuff the salad into the pita pockets and serve.

Pork Chop Milanese with Watercress and Blue Cheese Salad

the
BUSY
MOM'S
TIP

If you don't see pork cutlets in the meat section, ask your butcher for them. Every market has a butcher. Sometimes you just have to search him out.

■

You can buy toasted almonds, but it's easy to toast them yourself. Most of the toasted nuts sold in stores have added oils that just aren't necessary. Heat a sauté pan on low and add the almonds. Stirring occasionally, cook for 5 to 6 minutes, until golden brown.

Just like anyone else cooking meals for the family, I sometimes get stuck in a weekly routine of chicken and fish. My dad always reminds me to bring back the pork chop. This is his favorite dish, and the Pork Chop Sandwiches with Herbed Mayo (page 106) make great use of any leftovers.

FOR THE PORK CHOPS

¼ cup olive oil

8 boneless pork cutlets (see tip)

4 teaspoons salt

1 teaspoon black pepper

2 cups dried plain bread crumbs

3 tablespoons chopped Italian flat-leaf parsley

3 tablespoons chopped garlic

1 cup grated Parmigiano-Reggiano cheese

2 cups all-purpose flour

4 large eggs, beaten, in a medium bowl

FOR THE SALAD

3 large eggs

6 cups watercress

½ cup blue cheese crumbles

3 tablespoons slivered or shaved toasted almonds (see tip)

6 tablespoons extra-virgin olive oil (see tip, page 71)

2 tablespoons sherry vinegar or champagne vinegar

1 teaspoon salt

½ teaspoon black pepper

WHAT TO DO

FOR THE PORK CHOPS:

PREHEAT the oven to 450°F (see tip, page 91) and coat a baking sheet with the oil.

TO POUND THE CUTLETS FLAT, cover a cutting board with plastic wrap. Place the cutlets on top of the board and cover them with another sheet of plastic wrap. Use a mallet to flatten the cutlets. If you don't have a mallet, you can use the bottom of a small pot or the flat side of a large knife.

SEASON each cutlet with ½ teaspoon salt and ⅛ teaspoon black pepper.

IN A MEDIUM BOWL, combine the bread crumbs, parsley, garlic, and Parmesan.

MEASURE the flour into another medium bowl.

THE THREE-STEP BREADING PROCESS will require you to keep one hand dry and one wet, or you'll end up with a big mess. Line up your ingredients: pork chops, flour, eggs, bread crumb mixture.

USING THE HAND you'll keep dry, dredge a cutlet in flour, coating it on both sides. Let the excess flour fall off. Use your other hand to dip and coat the cutlet in the beaten eggs. Drop the cutlet in the bread crumb mixture and use your dry hand to completely coat the cutlet. Place the cutlet on the baking sheet and repeat the process until all the cutlets are breaded.

BAKE the cutlets for 12 to 15 minutes, until they're golden brown.

FOR THE SALAD:

IN A SMALL POT, cover the eggs with cold water and bring them to a boil. For hard-boiled eggs, let them simmer for 10 minutes. Let them cool in the fridge and then peel and quarter them.

IN A LARGE BOWL, combine the watercress, blue cheese, and almonds. Drizzle them with the extra-virgin olive oil and vinegar, and season with salt and pepper. Toss the salad to combine and top it with the eggs.

SERVE the Pork Chop Milanese with the salad. The breading on the cutlets is enough starch to round out the meal.

Pork Chop Sandwiches with Herbed Mayo

Here's a great use for leftover Pork Chop Milanese (page 104). The herbed mayonnaise adds fresh flavor to the sandwiches, but for non-mayo eaters, or for a healthier option, the mayonnaise can be replaced with mashed avocado.

6 tablespoons mayonnaise (or 1 whole avocado, mashed)

1 tablespoon chopped fresh chives

1 tablespoon chopped fresh tarragon

1 teaspoon champagne vinegar, white wine vinegar, or red wine vinegar

1 teaspoon chopped shallots

4 small Italian rolls (about 4 inches wide)

4 cooked pork cutlets

1 cup watercress

4 slices tomato

WHAT TO DO

IN A SMALL BOWL, combine the mayonnaise, chives, tarragon, vinegar, and shallots and blend well.

DRESS each side of the rolls with the mayonnaise. Lay a cutlet on one side and top it with watercress and tomato.

THIS IS A GREAT SANDWICH to pack for work, since it tastes great cold.

Movie Night

CARAMEL-ALMOND POPCORN

COCONUT MILK AND BANANA SMOOTHIE

CRUNCHY CASHEW BRITTLE

LEMON-PEPPER CHICKEN WINGS

FONDUE WITH GRUYÈRE AND FRESH FRUIT

A DUO OF CHIPS—KALE AND SWEET POTATO

SAUTÉED EDAMAME

GUACAMOLE AND TORTILLA CHIPS

I'M NORMALLY A BIG ADVOCATE OF TURNING OFF THE TELEVISION AND HAVING FAMily meals around the table. It's important to give one another that individual attention and actually have conversations, rather than staring at cartoon characters running across the screen while we eat. But movie nights are special. Friday evenings are our chance to rent videos, make fun foods, build a fort or snuggle on the couch, and bond over old memories while we create new ones.

My mom had movie nights with the kids when my dad worked late, and there was always fun food involved. I remember climbing in bed with her to watch movies while we ate cantaloupe and vanilla ice cream. My poor dad would come home to find my brother and me fast asleep, sprawled across his bed, and it was his job to carry us back to our rooms. It's the kind of simple, special memory every family creates, and the food makes it that much more memorable.

When Xea was born, I couldn't wait for her to be old enough to share the movies I'd enjoyed with my family growing up. *Clue*, *Troop Beverly Hills*, and *E.T.* were family favorites when I was a kid, and I've had so much fun sitting down with a great meal and sharing these movies with my daughter as she experienced them for the first time. I hope those nights are creating memories she'll one day share with her own kids.

The finger foods and snacks in this chapter will rival anything you'd get at the theater concession stand. They cost a lot less, and since you're making them, you'll know exactly what's going in them. I hope you'll make movie night with home-cooked treats a regular event at your house, too.

Caramel-Almond Popcorn

SERVES 4 to 6
TOTAL TIME: 30 minutes

Microwave popcorn has convinced us that cooking fresh popcorn is hard or time-consuming. It's not. You can do it on the stove top; it only takes a little oil and a few minutes. Just follow the package directions. Or you can always use microwave or premade plain popcorn in this recipe. *(see photo insert)*

1 cup light brown sugar, firmly packed
¼ cup light corn syrup
1 tablespoon salt
1 cup heavy cream, at room temperature
½ teaspoon vanilla extract
¼ teaspoon baking soda
8 cups popped popcorn
2 cups raw whole almonds

WHAT TO DO

COMBINE the sugar, corn syrup, and salt in a medium saucepot. Bring the mixture to a boil over medium heat and let it boil for 6 to 8 minutes without stirring. You have to watch it the whole time, because it will turn from sugar to caramel very quickly.

ONCE THE MIXTURE turns light brown, remove it from the heat and whisk in the cream. Stir in the vanilla and baking soda. Be careful not to touch the caramel until it has cooled. It will be scalding hot. Don't try to taste it!

SPREAD the popcorn and almonds in a large baking dish. Pour the caramel over them, using a plastic spatula to mix the popcorn and almonds. Make sure you stir from the bottom of the dish to coat everything well.

AS THE CARAMEL COOLS in the pan, stir a few more times to keep the caramel from sinking to the bottom of the dish. This popcorn is meant to be eaten the day it's made. If you need to save it for a few hours, simply cover it with parchment paper or a paper towel and leave it out on the countertop.

Coconut Milk and Banana Smoothie

This smoothie was inspired by my sister-in-law, who's always looking for the healthy version of everything. It's dairy-free and safe for those who have trouble with lactose. Best of all, it's like a dessert smoothie—but with better ingredients than most smoothies you get at the local stores. You can have this ready before the kids get through the previews on whichever movie you're watching.

3 cups coconut milk, unsweetened (see tip)
3 frozen bananas (see tip)
¼ teaspoon nutmeg
¼ teaspoon cinnamon
1 teaspoon vanilla extract
2 tablespoons honey

WHAT TO DO

POUR the coconut milk into the blender. Add the bananas, nutmeg, cinnamon, vanilla, and honey. Blend until smooth.

---

the BUSY MOM'S TIP

I like to use the cartons of coconut milk found in the refrigerated section of the supermarket. You can also use canned coconut milk, as long as it's unsweetened. Save the sweetened coconut milk for the grown-up smoothies, aka piña coladas.

If you have a high-speed blender, you can blend the frozen banana whole. If you have a conventional blender, break or slice the banana into thirds before you blend it, so it doesn't jam the blades.

Crunchy Cashew Brittle

MAKES about 10 servings

TOTAL TIME: 45 minutes

Cashews were a favorite of Xea's dad. His taste must have influenced me, because cashews are now my nut of choice. I think they make this brittle a little more special than your usual peanut brittle.

5 tablespoons cold unsalted butter

2 cups roasted unsalted cashews

1 cup sugar

¼ cup light corn syrup

¼ teaspoon salt

6 tablespoons water

WHAT TO DO

USE 2 tablespoons of the butter to grease a baking sheet and spread the cashews over it. Set the baking sheet aside.

IN A 2-QUART SAUCEPAN, heat the sugar, corn syrup, salt, and water on medium heat. Just as the sugar starts to dissolve, give it all one last stir with a wooden spoon. Let the mixture simmer until it reaches 295°F (see tip).

ADD the last 3 tablespoons of cold butter to the pot and stir it in.

POUR the syrup over the cashews and use a rubber spatula to make sure all the nuts are covered.

LET THE BRITTLE COOL for 20 to 25 minutes. Once the candy has completely cooled, snap it into pieces.

the
**BUSY
MOM'S
TIP**

You'll definitely need to use a candy thermometer to make this. The candy mixture will need to reach 295°F, and you can't eyeball that.

If you find the pot difficult to clean after you've cooked the brittle syrup, simply add 3 cups of water to the pot, bring it to a boil, and rinse it well.

Lemon-Pepper Chicken Wings

The beauty of the chicken wing is that even though it's white meat, it stays moist when you cook it. I like to roast wings in the oven and render the fat slowly. As the fat melts off, you get a crispy skin and tender meat that are as good as you get with fried chicken.

24 chicken wings (see tip)
6 tablespoons vegetable oil
¾ teaspoon salt
1 tablespoon Lawry's lemon-pepper seasoning (see tip)

WHAT TO DO

PREHEAT the oven to 450°F. Starting the cooking process at a high temperature will crisp the outside of the wings and seal in the juices.

PAT the wings dry and lay them on a large baking sheet. Pour the oil over the wings. Sprinkle the salt and lemon-pepper seasoning over the wings. Massage those ingredients into all of the wings, making sure to cover the wings completely on all sides.

SPREAD the wings out on the baking sheet, leaving at least ½ inch of space between them. If they're too close together, they'll steam instead of bake.

BAKE the wings for 12 to 15 minutes and then rotate the pan so that the wings at the back are moved to the front. Reduce the heat to 350°F. Bake for another 12 to 15 minutes, until golden brown, and remove the pan from the oven. Let the wings rest for 5 minutes. Serve with a salad.

the
**BUSY
MOM'S
TIP**

You can buy wings with the tips on or off, as you prefer. This recipe also works for drumettes that are usually used for buffalo wings.

◼

I don't take the time to measure out the lemon-pepper seasoning. I just use two big shakes of it on both sides of each wing. It's one of my favorite seasoning blends.

Fondue with Gruyère and Fresh Fruit

On *Top Chef All-Stars*, I was challenged to remake this 1970s classic. I came up with a fancy version involving smoked salmon, but that was for a competition. In my normal life, I still like this traditional take on fondue. In fact, Xea and I sometimes go to a local French restaurant to sit on the patio and share this simple meal.

3 tablespoons unsalted butter

1 tablespoon all-purpose flour

6 tablespoons kirsch or a sweet white wine

2 pounds Gruyère or a Swiss cheese, grated

¼ teaspoon nutmeg

¼ teaspoon black pepper

1 French baguette, cut into small chunks

6 servings of fresh fruit, such as apples, grapes, and strawberries (about 6 cups)

WHAT TO DO

IN A 2-QUART SACEPOT, melt the butter over medium-low heat. Whisk the flour into the melted butter and cook for 2 minutes. Whisk in the kirsch.

SLOWLY STIR in the cheese, a handful at a time. The cheese might have an occasional bubble as it melts, but it should never boil.

STIR in the nutmeg and pepper.

TRANSFER the fondue to a fondue pot (see tip). You can use whatever heating element comes with the fondue pot, but it isn't necessary if you're going to consume the fondue right away. Serve with a platter of bread and fruit.

the BUSY MOM'S TIP

You'll need a fondue pot to serve this dish. The pots are easy to find at discount stores and they aren't expensive. You can use the skewers that come with the fondue set, or pick up a pack of bamboo skewers to use instead. If you use bamboo, color the end of each skewer with a different colored marker, so each person knows which one is theirs.

A Duo of Chips—Kale and Sweet Potato

The first time I tried kale chips, I was with Xea, and she was sure they wouldn't taste good. The idea of a leaf as a chip was just weird. Turns out, we both loved them. They're addictive. It's amazing to look up and realize you've just eaten a whole bowl of kale.

FOR THE KALE CHIPS

2 bunches dinosaur kale (aka Lacinato kale)

6 tablespoons olive oil

¼ cup shredded Parmigiano-Reggiano cheese

FOR THE SWEET POTATO CHIPS

3 medium sweet potatoes, peeled

4 cups peanut or vegetable oil

¼ teaspoon salt

*1½ tablespoons chopped fresh sage or rosemary, or ¼ teaspoon
    dried sage or rosemary*

WHAT TO DO

FOR THE KALE CHIPS:

PREHEAT the oven to 300°F.

A FLAT KALE LEAF is easiest to work with. Slice the stems from the leaves and discard the stems. If you use curly kale, you should also remove the thick stem dividing each side of the leaf. Wash and dry the leaves.

BRUSH both sides of the leaves with the olive oil and spread them on two baking sheets. The leaves can be close together but shouldn't overlap.

SPRINKLE the leaves with the Parmesan. Bake for 20 to 25 minutes, until they're crispy but not overly brown.

REMOVE the kale chips from the baking sheets with a spatula and arrange them on one side of a large platter.

FOR THE SWEET POTATO CHIPS:

TRIM the ends from the peeled sweet potatoes and slice the potatoes into rounds ⅛ inch thick. The best tool for this job is a mandoline. (See the tip on page 19.) If you don't have a mandoline, use a sharp knife to slice the potatoes.

PREHEAT the peanut oil to 325°F, as measured by a candy thermometer, in a 3-quart pot or fryer (see tip, page 114). I prefer peanut oil because in addition to its light flavor, it has a very high smoke point, so it won't burn very easily. Vegetable or canola will also work.

RINSE the sliced potatoes under lukewarm water for about 2 minutes. This will remove the excess starch and keep the sweet potatoes from browning too much before they're cooked.

DRAIN the sweet potato slices in a colander and pat them dry with a paper towel. Divide them into 3 batches and fry them for 2½ to 3 minutes per batch (see tip, page 66). Keep rotating the chips as they cook to make sure they're covered and frying evenly.

PULL the potatoes out with a slotted spoon and drain them on a paper towel–lined plate. Sprinkle them with the salt and the chopped sage. Arrange the sweet potato chips on the platter next to the kale chips.

Sautéed Edamame

This warm dish combines salty and spicy flavors—perfect for movie-night snacking. *(see photo insert)*

¼ cup vegetable oil

1 (1-pound) bag of frozen precooked edamame, in the pod

3 tablespoons chopped pickled ginger

3 garlic cloves, chopped

2 teaspoons togarashi (optional; see tip)

1 cup ponzu sauce (see tip on this page and recipe on page 184)

2 scallions, chopped, for garnish

WHAT TO DO

POUR the oil into a 10-inch skillet. Add the edamame to the pan and heat the pan to medium high (see tip). Sauté the edamame for about 5 to 8 minutes. It should have a bit of color when it's done.

ADD the ginger, garlic, and togarashi to the pan and mix it in. Cook for about 1 minute to allow the flavors to bloom. Be careful not to burn the garlic!

STIR IN the ponzu sauce and cook for 2 more minutes.

TRANSFER the edamame to a serving bowl and garnish with the scallions.

the
**BUSY
MOM'S
TIP**

Togarashi is a Japanese pepper blend that can be found at most local supermarkets or specialty markets. If you can't find it, you can substitute chile flakes, or if you don't like your food spicy, you can just leave it out.

Ponzu sauce is a citrus-flavored soy sauce found with the Asian ingredients in most supermarkets.

I wouldn't normally add food to a cold pan, but since the edamame is frozen, adding it to a hot pan could cause oil to splatter.

Guacamole and Tortilla Chips

SERVES 6
TOTAL TIME: 10 minutes

We live in Los Angeles, where guacamole and chips is always a favorite snack. Sure, you can buy a bag of tortilla chips at any supermarket, but fresh chips taste so much better and they're easy to make.

FOR THE GUACAMOLE

3 avocados, diced (retain 1 pit; see tip)

½ medium yellow onion, diced into ⅛-inch pieces (see tip, page 49)

1 large tomato, cored, seeded, and diced into ⅛-inch pieces (see tip, page 30)

½ jalapeño pepper, finely diced

2 tablespoons chopped fresh cilantro

Juice of 1½ limes

½ teaspoon salt

FOR THE TORTILLA CHIPS

1 quart canola or vegetable oil, for frying

25 corn tortillas, cut into sixths

½ teaspoon salt

WHAT TO DO

FOR THE GUACAMOLE:

I LIKE MY GUACAMOLE CHUNKY, so I don't mash the avocados. They get slightly mashed as all the ingredients are stirred together.

COMBINE the avocados, onion, tomato, jalapeño, and cilantro in a medium bowl. Add the lime juice and salt. Stir all the ingredients to blend them together. Add the avocado pit to the mixture, leaving it in when you serve the dip.

the
**BUSY
MOM'S
TIP**

Leaving an avocado pit in the guacamole mixture will keep it from browning.

FOR THE TORTILLA CHIPS:

IN A DEEP FRYER or 4-quart pot on medium heat, heat the oil to 350°F, as measured by a candy thermometer. Add the chips to the hot oil, stirring continuously for 1 minute and turning the chips over with a slotted spoon. Cook the chips for 3 to 4 minutes, until they're golden brown (see tip, page 66). Remove the chips with a slotted spoon and set them to drain on a paper towel–lined plate. Sprinkle them with the salt and serve with the guacamole.

Family Style

EVERYTHING PAELLA

CRISPY CAULIFLOWER WITH PARMESAN

PIZZA WITH PROSCIUTTO AND BURRATA

MUSSELS AND FENNEL

GARLIC BREAD

CATFISH FRITTERS

SPICY CHICKEN GUMBO

PANZANELLA

BACON, BRUSSELS SPROUT, AND GOAT CHEESE PIE

GRILLED LAMB CHOPS WITH WATERMELON SALAD

MIXED BEAN SALAD WITH ROASTED BELL PEPPERS

MY PARENTS HOSTED BIG MEALS ALL THE TIME WHEN I WAS GROWING UP. With just our local extended family, we had a house filled with people, and friends were always welcome. Everyone would make a huge platter of one of the dishes she was famous for (no, the men weren't cooking for those events!), and we all had certain dishes we expected from each cook. I'd stand next to the stove waiting for the first, superhot taste of my mother's Crispy Cauliflower with Parmesan (page 123). The beauty of these events was that no one person was responsible for the whole meal. It's a low-stress way to feed a lot of people.

I still look forward to the energy of people from three or four generations laughing together and telling stories over a great meal. With my current work schedule, I don't get to do it as often as I'd like, but I love exposing Xea to that kind of interaction. It gives her the chance to learn how to communicate with people of all ages.

The dishes in this chapter lend themselves to serving large numbers of dinner guests, and most can be made, or at least started, the night before your event. They're also easily transportable, so taking them to someone else's house isn't a problem. If you don't have a big family to pull together for a meal, call your best friends and plan a potluck. Even if you do it only a few times a year, I promise it will bring you all a little closer together.

Everything Paella

Paella can look like an intimidating dish to make, but I don't want you to be scared of the ingredient list. I promise, if you have everything ready to go and work in an organized way, you'll be successful and you'll want to make this dish again and again.

the
BUSY MOM'S TIP

I recommend you invest in a 14- to 16-inch paella pan. Paellas need to be cooked and served in the same pan, because the rice will crisp nicely and you don't want to lose that while transferring to a platter. A paella pan is made to go from stove top to oven to table.

1 pound chicken drumettes

6 tablespoons, plus ¼ cup vegetable oil

¾ teaspoon salt, plus more to taste

½ teaspoon black pepper, plus more to taste

1 pound manila clams, black mussels, or a mix of both

1 pound 16/20-count shrimp, peeled and deveined, tail-on (frozen is fine, see tip, page 58)

½ pound fresh chorizo cut into 1-inch cubes or ¼ pound dried chorizo cut into ½-inch cubes

1 medium red bell pepper, sliced into ⅛-inch strips

1 medium green bell pepper, sliced into ⅛-inch strips

1 medium yellow onion, sliced ⅛-inch thick

2 teaspoons chicken Better Than Bouillon or 2 bouillon cubes

6 cups water

3 cups Uncle Ben's parboiled rice

2 teaspoons saffron

⅓ cup chopped fresh cilantro

WHAT TO DO

PREHEAT the oven to 450°F (see tip, page 91).

SPREAD the drumettes on a baking sheet and drizzle them with the 6 tablespoons vegetable oil. Season them with ¼ teaspoon salt and ¼ teaspoon black pepper and rub the oil and seasonings into the drumettes. Roast for 15 minutes, just until they're crispy. Remove the chicken from the oven and set it aside. Leave the oven on.

WHILE THE DRUMETTES ARE COOKING, clean the clams and/or mussels. The mussels have a visible beard that needs to be removed. You can just use your fingers to pull the hairs off as you're washing the mussels. Place the mussels and clams in the bottom of the sink under cold running water. If any of them are open and don't close under the cold water, they're dead and need to be discarded. Mussels and clams tend to be sandy; knock them around against one another under the running water to clear away any sand. You don't want grit in your paella.

IN YOUR PAELLA PAN (see tip), heat the ¼ cup of vegetable oil on medium heat. Add the chorizo and brown it in the oil. Add the peppers and onion and season with ¼ teaspoon salt and ¼ teaspoon pepper. Cook until the vegetables soften and take on a little color.

DISSOLVE the bouillon in 1 cup of water.

ADD the rice, Better Than Bouillon, 5 cups more water, and saffron to the pan. Give everything a stir to mix it, but don't stir it too much. Your rice will release too much starch and become mushy with too much stirring—you don't want mushy rice in your paella.

REDUCE the heat to low and flatten out the mixture in the pan. Place the chicken, mussels, clams, and shrimp on top of the rice. Season it all with a pinch of salt.

COVER the pan and cook for 12 to 15 minutes, until the rice is cooked. As soon as the rice is cooked, turn up the heat to high and cook for 1 minute more.

UNCOVER the pan and pop it in the oven. Let the paella bake for 10 minutes. The mussels and/or clams should have opened and the rice should be slightly crispy and turning golden brown.

SPRINKLE the paella with the chopped cilantro and serve.

Crispy Cauliflower with Parmesan

My mother taught me how to make this when I was a kid. I always loved it, and I always thought it belonged on a restaurant menu. Recently my parents came to my restaurant and ordered this dish. They loved it, and my mother asked me for the recipe! Mom, it's your recipe.

2 quarts vegetable oil

3 cups shredded Parmigiano-Reggiano

12 large eggs, beaten

6 cups all-purpose flour

2 tablespoons salt

3 heads of cauliflower, broken into medium florets

Grated zest of 3 lemons, to garnish

¾ cup shredded Parmigiano-Reggiano cheese, to garnish

3 tablespoons chopped Italian flat-leaf parsley, to garnish

lemon wedges (optional)

the
**BUSY
MOM'S
TIP**

If you like, you can serve with lemon wedges. Anyone who wants to can squeeze lemon juice over their portion.

WHAT TO DO

IN A SMALL DEEP FRYER or 4- to 5-quart pot, heat the oil to 350°F, as verified by a candy thermometer (see tip, page 76).

IN A MEDIUM BOWL, combine the 3 cups Parmigiano-Reggiano and the beaten eggs.

IN A SEPARATE BOWL, combine the flour and salt.

USING YOUR FINGERS, dip the cauliflower florets into the egg mixture and then into the flour mixture.

WORKING IN BATCHES so the deep fryer isn't too crowded, fry the florets for 3 to 4 minutes, until they're golden brown (see tip, page 66). Drain them on a paper towel–covered plate.

ARRANGE the florets on a platter and garnish with the lemon zest, Parmigiano-Reggiano, and parsley.

Pizza with Prosciutto and Burrata

Pizza dough is easy to make, but a lot of pizza restaurants will sell their dough for you to take home. Or you can buy dough at your local supermarket. *(see photo insert)*

FOR THE DOUGH

3 cups all-purpose flour, plus more for rolling

1 tablespoon sugar

1 teaspoon salt

1 package active dry yeast

3 tablespoons olive oil

1½ cups lukewarm water

FOR THE PIZZA

2 tablespoons olive oil

¾ cup shredded low-moisture whole-milk mozzarella cheese

2 Roma tomatoes, cut into 8 slices each (see tip, page 67)

¼ teaspoon salt

Dash black pepper (just a sprinkle)

8 thin slices prosciutto

½ pound burrata (see tip)

1 tablespoon extra-virgin olive oil

1 tablespoon balsamic vinegar or balsamic reduction

4 large fresh basil leaves, thinly sliced

WHAT TO DO

FOR THE DOUGH:

MEASURE the flour, sugar, and salt into a food processor. (If you don't have a food processor, combine the flour, sugar, and salt in a large bowl and use your fingers to make a well in the center of the mixture.)

the
**BUSY
MOM'S
TIP**

Burrata is a type of mozzarella cheese. It's softer and richer than the typical mozzarella, because the milk solids aren't cooked as much. You can find it in many of the larger supermarket chains, in specialty markets, or online. Don't ever be limited by the fact that you can't find a special ingredient at your local store. No matter how small your town is, you can find any ingredient, even the most exotic, by shopping online.

STIR the yeast and olive oil into the lukewarm water. I like to measure the water in a 2-cup measuring cup and just add ingredients to it, rather than dirty another bowl.

TURN the food processor on low and stream in the liquid mixture. Let it spin for about a minute, or until the dough forms a ball. (If you're using your hands, pour the liquid mixture into the well of the dry ingredients. Use your fingertips to work the dry ingredients into the liquid, kneading for about 4 minutes, or until you have a ball of dough.)

PLACE the ball of dough on a plate and cover it with a clean, wet dish towel. Let it rest in the refrigerator for 40 minutes. It should be about a quarter larger in size when it's ready to roll out.

FOR THE PIZZA:

PREHEAT the oven to 425°F (see tip, page 91). If you have a convection oven, use it but reduce the temperature to 375°F.

ROLL OUT the dough on a dry, lightly floured surface. If you don't have a rolling pin, you can even use an empty wine bottle. To roll the dough for a circular pan, take your rolling pin and press it down in the center of the dough, rolling upward, downward, and to the right 1½ inches. Turn the dough a quarter turn and repeat that process all the way around to make a circle. The dough should be 12 to 14 inches wide and ¼ inch thick when you're done.

TO MOVE THE DOUGH TO THE PAN, you'll use the rolling pin again. Start at the bottom of the dough and roll it over the pin, as if you were curling someone's hair. You want to end with the whole dough wrapped around your pin. Roll the pin over the pizza pan, allowing the dough to unfold over the pan. Now you need to clock the dough to prevent air bubbles. Use a fork (or even your fingernails) to pierce tiny holes all over the dough.

WITH A PASTRY BRUSH, spread 2 tablespoons olive oil over the surface of the dough. Sprinkle the shredded mozzarella over the dough and top it with the tomato slices. Season the tomatoes with the salt and pepper. Bake the pizza for 12 to 15 minutes, rotating it a quarter turn every 4 minutes.

the
**BUSY
MOM'S
TIP**

If you want to invest in a pizza stone, I highly recommend them. You can use them to cook and to serve your pizza and it will give you the best texture, closest to what you'd get from a brick oven. Or you can just use a round pizza pan, or even a rectangular baking sheet.

ONCE THE CHEESE IS MELTED and the edges of the crust are crispy, remove the pizza from the oven and let it rest for about 2 minutes. Slice the pizza into 8 pieces. You want to slice it before you add the prosciutto, because the meat can be difficult to cut and would likely cause you to rip the cheese and bread while you tried to slice it.

LIGHTLY LAY a slice of prosciutto on each slice of pizza. Add a dollop of burrata on each piece of prosciutto, using the entire ½ pound.

DRIZZLE the pizza with 1 tablespoon extra-virgin olive oil and the balsamic vinegar to dress the burrata and prosciutto. Garnish with the thinly sliced basil.

Mussels and Fennel

SERVES 10 to 12
TOTAL TIME: 20 minutes

When I made mussels on *Top Chef All-Stars*, I was terrified. I kept thinking my mussels weren't cleaned well enough, and the worst thing you can do is serve gritty mussels. I ended up winning an Elimination Challenge with a dish like this, so I guess I'd done a better job cleaning the mussels than I thought. The lesson: clean your mussels well. And then clean them again! *(see photo insert)*

the
**BUSY
MOM'S
TIP**

4 sticks (1 pound) unsalted butter

1 bulb fennel, thinly shaved with a mandoline (see tip, page 19)

¼ teaspoon red pepper flakes

2 sprigs of fresh tarragon

2 sprigs of fresh rosemary

2 sprigs of fresh thyme

8 garlic cloves, chopped

5 pounds mussels, well cleaned (see tip)

½ teaspoon salt

⅓ cup sugar

3 cups dry white wine (see tip, page 128)

¼ cup chopped Italian flat-leaf parsley

1 baguette, sliced and toasted in the oven

To clean the mussels, put them in the sink under cold running water. Move them around with your hands, so they're bumping against one another. This will help knock away any sand, so you won't end up with grit in your dish. Rinse the mussels well and use your fingers to tear away the beard on each one. As they're exposed to the cold water, any open mussels should close. If they don't, they're dead and you should throw them out. Discard any mussels with cracked shells as well.

WHAT TO DO

IN A LARGE SHALLOW POT 14 to 16 inches wide, melt the butter over medium heat. Add the shaved fennel, red pepper flakes, tarragon, rosemary, thyme, and garlic. Cook for 4 minutes.

THROW IN the mussels and season with the salt. Add the sugar to the pan and turn the mussels over to coat them.

Some chefs claim you need to use fancy, expensive wine for cooking. I think it's unnecessary. An inexpensive white wine, like a dry Chablis, will be just as good for cooking as a more expensive one.

If you have any open wine bottles in your fridge, just use what you have. Make sure you taste the wine before you use it, making sure it hasn't turned.

POUR the wine over the mussels and let everything cook for about 5 minutes, or until the mussels open. The broth should cook down so there's no taste of alcohol left from the wine.

TURN OUT the mussels and broth into a large, family-style bowl. Leave the whole herbs in for garnish and spread the fennel evenly over the dish.

GARNISH the dish with the chopped parsley and stick the toasted bread around the sides of the bowl.

Garlic Bread

Who doesn't love crunchy, buttery garlic bread? This is great for dipping in the broth of Mussels and Fennel (page 127).

2 whole garlic cloves
1 stick (½ cup) unsalted butter, softened
¼ teaspoon salt
2 tablespoons chopped Italian flat-leaf parsley
2 large loaves Italian bread

WHAT TO DO

PREHEAT the broiler to high.

WITH THE FLAT SIDE OF A KNIFE, smash the cloves of garlic on a cutting board. Chop the garlic to death. (If you have a garlic press, you can peel the cloves and press them. I prefer to use my knife, but use what's easiest for you.)

IN A SMALL BOWL, whip the garlic into the softened butter with the salt. Mix in the parsley.

SLICE the loaves in half lengthwise. Cut those two pieces in half and place them on a baking sheet. Toast the bread under the broiler on high until crisp. Remove the bread from the oven and spread garlic butter over each piece.

PUT the bread back under the broiler for another 45 seconds to 1 minute to warm the garlic. Slice and serve.

the
**BUSY
MOM'S
TIP**

The broiler cooks so fast, you might want to stand there and watch it so the bread doesn't burn. I usually leave the oven door open to remind myself to keep a close eye on it, but keep the kids out of the kitchen if you use this reminder.

Catfish Fritters

The Wondra flour used in this recipe is a brand of finely milled flour that's great for breading. It distills the usual three-step breading process into one step, saves time, and reduces cleanup. You can find it in most major supermarkets or order it online.

When I was twenty years old, I moved to New York City to start culinary school. My first job was waiting tables and managing Justin's Restaurant for Sean "Puffy" Combs. It was the first time I'd ever tried soul food. The restaurant introduced me to Southern classics such as collards, smothered turkey wings, and red velvet cake. It was also my introduction to catfish, and I was obsessed with these fritters from the first bite. I couldn't believe I'd spent my whole life deprived of this whole other culture of food.

1 quart peanut oil or canola oil

½ cup hot sauce (I like Louisiana Crystal, but use your favorite)

2 cups mayonnaise

3 pounds skinless, boneless catfish fillets

¼ cup Lawry's seasoned salt

2 cups Wondra flour (see tip)

4 lemons, cut into wedges

WHAT TO DO

ADD the oil to a 4-quart saucepot or your deep fryer and heat to 400°F, verifying the temperature with a candy thermometer (see tip, page 76).

COMBINE the hot sauce and mayonnaise in a small bowl and set it aside.

SLICE the fillets in the shape of small chicken fingers. They should be about 1½ inches long and ½ inch wide. You want them to be about two bites each, maybe one bite if you're a guy.

SEASON the fillets generously with the seasoned salt.

PUT the Wondra flour in a medium bowl. Drop the catfish pieces into the flour a few at a time, shaking the bowl to cover the catfish with the flour. As you remove each piece, give it a shake to remove any excess flour and set it aside on a plate.

FRY the catfish fritters for 2 to 3 minutes, until they're golden brown (see tip, page 66). Use a slotted spoon to transfer them to a paper towel–lined plate to drain.

PUT the fritters on a platter, garnish with lemon wedges, and serve with the bowl of sauce in the center.

Spicy Chicken Gumbo

The filé powder used in gumbo is a classic ingredient in Cajun and Creole cooking. It's made from the powdered leaves of the sassafras tree, and it adds a unique, earthy flavor that you can't get from anything else.

You don't need to use expensive lump crabmeat or Alaskan king crab for this dish. Blue crab is typical of New Orleans, but any good-quality canned crabmeat will add the flavor you want. It will just break up in the stew anyway, so you don't need to pay for premium crabmeat.

1 pound chicken drumettes

1 teaspoon salt

¼ teaspoon black pepper

6 tablespoons, plus ¼ cup vegetable oil

2 medium yellow onions, diced

1 jalapeño pepper, roughly chopped, with seeds

1 large red bell pepper, cored, seeded, and diced

1 large green bell pepper, cored, seeded, and diced

1 pound chicken andouille sausage

1 cup all-purpose flour

1 tablespoon chicken Better Than Bouillon or 3 bouillon cubes

12 cups water

4 Roma tomatoes, roughly chopped

6 cobs of corn, kernels sliced off (see tip, page 60)

1 (28-ounce) can of crushed tomatoes

2 cups okra, sliced into ringlets

1 tablespoon Lawry's lemon-pepper seasoning

1½ cups crabmeat, picked over (see tip)

1 tablespoon filé powder

8 cups cooked white rice or a crispy baguette, for serving

WHAT TO DO

PREHEAT the oven to 425°F (see tip, page 91).

YOU'LL ROAST THE DRUMETTES before you add them to the gumbo. Spread them on a baking sheet and season them with a pinch of salt and a ⅛ teaspoon black pepper. Rub the chicken with the 6 tablespoons of vegetable oil, and roast for 15 minutes, or until the drumettes are crispy. Set aside the chicken to be added to the gumbo near the end of cooking.

IN A 6-QUART SAUCEPOT, heat the ¼ cup vegetable oil over medium heat. Add the onions, jalapeño, and red and green bell peppers, and season with ½ teaspoon salt and ⅛ teaspoon pepper. Add the andouille sausage, and cook it all over medium heat for 4 to 5 minutes, stirring occasionally, until the vegetables soften. You don't want to brown the vegetables, just allow them to cook down.

ADD the flour and stir it into the oil. Continue stirring, letting the flour absorb the excess oil. If you find it's sticking, you can add a bit more oil. You want to keep cooking until the sauce develops a nice brown color. This is the roux, and it thickens the gumbo.

ONCE YOUR ROUX IS BROWNED, add the bouillon cubes and the water to the pot. Add the Roma tomatoes, corn, crushed tomatoes, and okra, and reduce the heat to low. Stir in the lemon-pepper seasoning and let the pot simmer for 15 minutes.

ADD the drumettes to the gumbo and simmer for 5 more minutes. Stir in the crabmeat and filé powder and remove the gumbo from the heat. Serve over white rice or with a crispy baguette.

Panzanella

When I was a kid, my dad always ate his salad at the end of his meal, and always with bread. The bread was almost like another utensil and it would end up becoming a part of the salad. Later, I realized that the refined bread salad I saw in Italian restaurants was really just a take on this peasant-style way of eating.

FOR THE RICOTTA CHEESE

6 cups whole milk

6 ounces (¾ cup) heavy cream

6 ounces (¾ cup) low-fat plain yogurt

¼ teaspoon salt

Dash nutmeg

FOR THE PANZANELLA

½ cup olive oil

1 loaf Italian baguette, sliced on the bias into 12 slices

2 cups cherry tomatoes, cut in half

¼ cup green Italian olives, pitted and sliced

2 cups arugula

8 large fresh basil leaves, torn

⅓ cup extra-virgin olive oil (see tip, page 71)

¼ cup sherry vinegar

¼ teaspoon salt

¼ teaspoon black pepper

1 cup ricotta cheese (from above)

WHAT TO DO

FOR THE RICOTTA:

IN A 2-QUART SAUCEPOT over medium heat, whisk together the milk, heavy cream, yogurt, salt, and nutmeg. A word of warning: you don't want this mixture to boil

I highly recommend making your own ricotta to go with this Italian bread salad. It's a mildly flavored cheese, but the store-bought tends to be almost tasteless. The homemade ricotta is easy to make and much more flavorful; it can be made up to two days in advance.

at all. Keep an eye on it—if it threatens to boil, reduce the heat. Simmer for 15 to 20 minutes.

THE MILK SOLIDS will separate from the liquid and form a raft floating on top. Remove the pot from the heat and strain the mixture through a cheesecloth.

TIE TWO DIAGONAL CORNERS OF THE CLOTH in a firm knot over the remaining solids. Tie the other two diagonal corners in another knot over the first one. You want the cheese to continue to drain as it cools. An easy way to accomplish this is to secure the cheesecloth to a long spoon handle and lay the spoon across a large bowl so the cheese is suspended over the bowl and continues to drain. It should look like the "hobo bundle" kids make when they're threatening to run away from home. Let the ricotta cool in the fridge.

FOR THE PANZANELLA:
IN A 10-INCH SAUTÉ PAN, heat ½ cup of the olive oil over medium heat. You don't want to burn the oil, so reduce the heat if you notice any smoking. Working in batches, toast the slices of baguette in the pan on both sides. They should be golden brown.

IN A MEDIUM BOWL, combine the tomatoes, olives, arugula, and basil. Dress them with the ⅓ cup extra-virgin olive oil and the sherry vinegar. Season with salt and pepper and toss well.

ARRANGE the toasted bread on a platter. Top it with the salad mixture. Crumble the ricotta cheese on top and serve.

the
BUSY
MOM'S
TIP

The homemade piecrust I use for this dish has only four ingredients, and one of them is water. How simple is that? You can even make the crust a day before making the pie. It'll keep in the fridge for a day or in the freezer for up to six months. If you want to save even more time on the day of your event, you can cook the ingredients, let them cool, assemble the pie, cover it with a layer of plastic wrap and a layer of aluminum foil, and freeze it. It will keep for up to six months. When you're ready to serve, just bake it at 350°F for an hour and 15 minutes. It goes straight from the freezer to the oven.

Bacon, Brussels Sprout, and Goat Cheese Pie

I came up with this dish when I was doing my "Don't Be Afraid of the Crust" pie-making demonstration at Xea's school. People treat piecrust as the test of a good cook—if you make your own, you're actually cooking, and if not, you cheated. I don't begrudge anyone the use of a ready-made crust. I just want people to know homemade piecrust is easy to make.

FOR THE PIECRUST

2 sticks (1 cup) cold unsalted butter, cubed

2 cups all-purpose flour, plus more for rolling

1 tablespoon salt

½ cup ice water

FOR THE PIE

2 tablespoons vegetable oil

1 pound smoked bacon, cut into ¼-inch pieces

1 pound Brussels sprouts, stems removed and quartered

¼ teaspoon salt

1 piecrust (from above)

½ cup shredded fontina cheese

½ cup shredded mozzarella cheese

¼ cup crumbled goat cheese

WHAT TO DO

FOR THE PIECRUST:

COMBINE the butter, flour, and salt in a food processor; pulse for 1 minute. Once the butter has been chopped, set the processor to spin and drizzle in the ice water. You want to blend it for no more than 45 seconds. The dough should form a ball in the food processor.

REMOVE the dough, flatten it like a Frisbee, and wrap it in plastic. Let it rest in the fridge for at least 20 minutes, or up to a day.

FOR THE PIE:

PREHEAT the oven to 350°F.

IN A 10- TO 12-INCH SAUTÉ PAN over medium heat, heat the 2 tablespoons vegetable oil. Add the chopped bacon and cook until slightly crispy.

ONCE THE BACON IS CRISPY, remove it from the pan. Add the Brussels sprouts to the pan and season them with the salt. Cook the Brussels sprouts in the bacon fat and oil for 4 to 6 minutes, until golden brown and soft. Strain to remove the excess oil; otherwise the pie dough will become soggy when you add the filling. Transfer the Brussels sprouts to the plate where you have the bacon and let the bacon and Brussels sprouts cool in the fridge while you prepare the dough.

IF THE DOUGH has been in the fridge for a while, give it a few minutes to warm up. On a dry, lightly floured surface, press your rolling pin down in the dough, rolling upward, downward. Turn the dough a quarter turn and repeat that process all the way around to make a nice circular shape. You want to have about 2 inches of crust overhanging your pie pan.

ROLL the crust onto the pin, so the whole crust can be moved at once. Gently roll the pin across the pie pan, leaving the crust behind. Once the crust is arranged in the pie pan, roll the pin across the ridge of the pan. This will cut off the excess crust and leave a clean edge.

IN A MEDIUM BOWL, combine the fontina and mozzarella cheeses.

LAYER half of the cheese on the crust. Top it with the bacon and Brussels sprouts. Layer on the rest of the mixed cheeses. The Brussels sprouts should be completely covered, so they won't continue to brown. Sprinkle on the goat cheese.

BAKE the pie for 45 minutes, rotating it halfway through the baking time. The pie will be a beautiful golden brown. Serve warm or at room temperature.

Grilled Lamb Chops with Watermelon Salad

If you don't have a grill, you can cook these lamb chops under a broiler set to high for 3 minutes on each side. Like most chefs, I usually like meat cooked medium rare, but lamb is one exception to this rule. I tend to serve it cooked medium. The only way to perfect the art of cooking meat to your preferred temperature is to do it over and over again, so don't be afraid to try it.

For me, lamb chops symbolize a turning point in my parents' lives. When they were newly married and living on Long Island, they didn't make much money and really couldn't afford to take us out to eat. In the eighties, we moved to Las Vegas, where things were booming. They were finally making enough money to take us out to real restaurants, where my brother would always order lamb chops. They were proud to be able to provide for their family in that way, and proud that their young son would eat such a sophisticated dish. *(see photo insert)*

12 to 16 lamb chops

1 teaspoon salt

¼ teaspoon black pepper

2 tablespoons olive oil

½ medium watermelon, seeded and cut into 1-inch cubes

3 tablespoons capers, drained

4 tablespoons fresh chopped mint

2 tablespoons pitted, chopped kalamata olives

1 medium hothouse cucumber, sliced

3 tablespoons crumbled feta cheese

3 tablespoons extra-virgin olive oil, for dressing

1 tablespoon sherry vinegar

2 cups baby spinach

WHAT TO DO

HEAT the grill to medium (see tip) and season the lamb chops with the salt and pepper. Drizzle 2 tablespoons of the olive oil over the chops and rub it in with your hands. Grill the lamb chops for 3 minutes per side for 1-inch-thick chops, or 4 minutes per side for 2-inch-thick chops. Remove them from the grill and let them rest for 10 minutes.

IN A LARGE BOWL, combine the watermelon, the capers, 2 tablespoons of the mint, and the olives, cucumber, and feta cheese. Drizzle the extra-virgin olive oil and vinegar over the salad, tossing it well. Toss in the baby spinach.

SPOON the salad into the middle of a large platter. Arrange the lamb chops so they're standing around the salad. Garnish the platter with the remaining 2 tablespoons of mint and serve.

Mixed Bean Salad with Roasted Bell Peppers

SERVES 6 to 8
TOTAL TIME: 30 minutes

This bean salad keeps well overnight in the refrigerator, so you can make it the night before your event. Add the meat and cheese just before serving.

◾

If you want to use canned roasted red bell peppers you can. But promise me you'll try to roast you own at some point. It's really easy.

This recipe came out of a *Top Chef* challenge. Our mission: run door to door and raid neighborhood pantries to make a dish for a huge block party. I stumbled on a house with cans and cans of beans stashed under the kitchen sink. It was strange, but the result was this simple and satisfying bean salad.

3 large yellow bell peppers

1 pound green beans

4 cups water

2 teaspoons salt

2 cups ice water

5 (15.5-ounce) cans of beans (any mix of black, kidney, northern, pinto, or white kidney beans)

2 tablespoons chopped fresh oregano

Dash salt

Dash black pepper

2 tablespoons balsamic vinegar

¼ cup extra-virgin olive oil (see tip, page 71)

1 pound salami, cut into ½-inch-wide strips

1 pound prosciutto, cut into ½-inch-wide strips

1 cup crumbled diced provolone cheese

WHAT TO DO

ROAST the bell peppers. This might sound intimidating, but it's really simple (see tip). Place the peppers either on the open flame of a gas burner or on a grill set to medium-high heat. With metal tongs, rotate the peppers so that each side starts to soften and wilt.

ONCE THE PEPPERS ARE SOFT and charred, put them together in a large bowl and cover it tightly with plastic wrap, so no air escapes. Let them steam in the bowl for about 15 minutes. The steam makes them much easier to peel.

PEEL, core, seed, and dice the peppers. If you have trouble removing the skins, run the peppers under just a bit of water. This is a rustic salad, so don't worry about any skin that's left behind.

CLEAN the green beans and cut them into pieces about the size of the other beans. Bring the 4 cups of water to a boil and add the 2 teaspoons of salt to it. Drop the green beans in for about 1½ minutes to blanch them. They should be bright green.

USING A SLOTTED SPOON, remove the green beans from the pot and drop them in a bowl with the 2 cups ice water. This will stop the cooking process and help them retain their color and crunchiness.

EMPTY all the canned beans into a colander. Rinse and drain them well.

IN A LARGE BOWL, combine the diced yellow peppers, blanched green beans, mixed canned beans, and half of the chopped oregano. Season with a dash each of salt and pepper. Mix in the balsamic vinegar and extra-virgin olive oil.

SPOON the mixed bean salad into the middle of a large serving platter. Arrange the salami and prosciutto around the salad. Top the meat with diced provolone cheese. Loosely sprinkle the remaining oregano over the cheese.

Sunday Dinner

TEX-MEX TURKEY CHILI

HONEY CORN CAKES

BARBECUE PULLED-PORK SANDWICHES

FRESH CABBAGE SLAW

BREAD-AND-BUTTER PICKLES

GRANDMA'S LASAGNA

OLD-FASHIONED POT ROAST

ROSEMARY MASHED POTATOES

SPAGHETTI AND MEATBALLS

ESCAROLE SALAD

CRISPY FRIED CHICKEN

WARM MUSHROOM SALAD WITH POACHED EGGS
AND BACON VINAIGRETTE

BONE-IN RIB EYE WITH SAUCE

ROASTED FENNEL AND CIPOLLINI

SHALLOT-POTATO GRATIN

WHEN I WAS A KID, SUNDAY DINNER WAS ALWAYS A TIME FOR THE EXTENDED family to come together. Dinner started at four in the afternoon and lasted until eight at night. Imagine all the intimate chaos of the holidays on a smaller scale—the smell of sauce cooking on the stove, the energy of kids running around the house, and the noise of aunts and uncles, parents and grandparents, all talking at the same time. Each of the women had a hand in the cooking (while the men sat around in their undershirts), and all the adults told stories about their past and talked about what was going on in their lives.

As a kid fighting for my place in those conversations, I learned how to communicate with people of all ages and how to stand up for myself and express my opinion. I also learned a lot of social skills, including when to respect my elders and keep my mouth shut!

When we all get together these days, my parents take a backseat to our generation while the grandkids listen to stories about our childhood, and conversations about all the things we have going on now: parenting, relationships, managing careers and businesses. We've become the keepers of the family history, and it's our job to share it with the next generation.

Sometimes a Sunday dinner is just Xea and me, and we talk about our week. Those nights are quieter, but just as important. Occasionally we invite a few girlfriends and Xea gets to see me in my role as a woman and a friend, not just as a mother.

You don't need to gather with a huge family to linger over a leisurely Sunday dinner. The following indulgent, comforting recipes may take a little more time than usual, but they provide a great opportunity to slow down and enjoy the process of cooking. The final products invite you to stay at the table and laugh and talk together, whether you're a party of two or twenty.

Tex-Mex Turkey Chili

Most people serve chili with shredded cheddar cheese. Cheddar is always good, but for a more traditional Tex-Mex flavor, try *cotija* cheese. This hard Mexican cheese shreds or crumbles nicely.

¼ cup vegetable oil

1 pound ground turkey (dark or white meat, or a mixture of both; see tip)

1 tablespoon salt

1 small red bell pepper, diced ½ inch thick (see tip, page 49)

1 small green bell pepper, diced ½ inch thick

1 small yellow onion, diced ½ inch thick

1 teaspoon crushed chipotle pepper

2 tablespoons ground coriander

2 tablespoons ground cumin

1 teaspoon smoked paprika

1 (28-ounce) can of crushed tomatoes

¼ cup molasses

¼ cup apple cider vinegar

¼ cup light brown sugar, firmly packed

1½ cups chicken stock, or equivalent Better Than Bouillon or bouillon cubes
    (see tip, page 51)

1 (15.5-ounce) can of black beans

15 ounces corn (fresh, frozen, or canned)

OPTIONAL TOPPINGS

Sour cream

Chopped fresh chives

Chopped green onion

Shredded cheese (such as queso fresco, Monterey Jack, cheddar, or cotija)

Sliced avocado

the
**BUSY
MOM'S
TIP**

Because there's so much liquid in this dish, you can use all-white-meat turkey for a lower-fat option. The chili is so flavorful, you won't miss the fat.

WHAT TO DO

IN A 4-QUART SAUCEPAN, heat the vegetable oil on high heat. Brown the ground turkey with the salt until it's cooked through. Add the bell peppers and onion and cook for another 3 minutes.

STIR IN THE DRIED CHIPOTLE, coriander, cumin, and paprika. Cook for another 2 to 3 minutes to bloom the spices, bringing out their full flavor and fragrance.

ADD the tomatoes, molasses, vinegar, brown sugar, and chicken stock. Reduce the heat to medium-low and let the chili simmer for 15 minutes.

STIR IN the black beans and corn. Simmer for another 5 minutes.

SERVE with the toppings your family will enjoy. Honey Corn Cakes (page 147) are also a favorite with chili, and the cakes can be baked while the chili simmers.

Honey Corn Cakes

These corn cakes are made mostly of the nonperishable ingredients you probably already have in your cabinets. They're easy to make and go great with chili, soup, or breakfast.

1½ cups all-purpose flour

½ cup cornmeal

⅓ cup sugar

1 tablespoon baking powder

1 teaspoon salt

1¼ cups buttermilk

2 large eggs

⅓ cup vegetable oil

6 tablespoons unsalted butter, melted

1 (11-ounce) can of corn, drained

Nonstick vegetable oil spray

⅓ cup honey

WHAT TO DO

PREHEAT the oven to 350°F.

IN A LARGE BOWL, combine the flour, cornmeal, sugar, baking powder, and salt.

IN A MEDIUM BOWL or 4-cup measuring cup, combine the buttermilk, eggs, and oil and whisk well.

POUR the wet ingredients into the dry ingredients and stir until they're well combined. Fold the melted butter into the batter. Fold in the canned corn.

GREASE two muffin tins with vegetable oil spray. Use a 2-ounce ice cream scoop to pour equal portions of the batter into the tins (see tip).

> *the* **BUSY MOM'S TIP**
>
> Baking individual cakes in a muffin tin, instead of baking one large loaf, helps you create the perfect portion sizes.

BAKE the corn cakes for 14 minutes, or until they're firm to touch. Remove them from the oven and use a toothpick to poke 10 to 12 holes in each corn cake.

USE a pastry brush to brush each corn cake with honey. The honey will be absorbed into each cake.

Barbecue Pulled-Pork Sandwiches

MAKES 10 to 12 sandwiches
PREP TIME: 35 minutes
COOKING TIME: 2½ to
5 hours

My friends who've made this recipe say it ruined restaurant pulled pork for them. Their old favorite just can't compete with these layered flavors. I even had my sixty-two-year-old retired construction worker dad test this out, and he was amazed at what he'd cooked. These sandwiches are great topped with Fresh Cabbage Slaw (page 151) and served with a side of Bread-and-Butter Pickles (page 152).

FOR THE SPICE RUB

2 tablespoons smoked paprika

2 tablespoons garlic powder

2 tablespoons onion powder

¼ teaspoon black pepper

¼ cup salt

2 tablespoons ground coffee beans

FOR THE PORK AND SAUCE

4 pounds boneless pork butt, cut into 3 pieces of equal size

6 tablespoons vegetable or canola oil

2 cups bourbon, whiskey, or scotch

3 cups chicken stock, or equivalent Better Than Bouillon (see tip, page 51)

1 (18-ounce) bottle of barbecue sauce (use your favorite)

2 tablespoons apple cider vinegar

1 cup light brown sugar, firmly packed

¼ cup molasses

10 to 12 Hawaiian bread buns, French rolls, or hamburger rolls (about 4–6 inches wide)

2 stalks green onion, including whites, chopped, for garnish

the
**BUSY
MOM'S
TIP**

If you don't have a Crock-Pot, the pork can be cooked for 2½ to 3 hours simmering on a low temperature in a covered stewing pot. If you have a pressure cooker, you can use it to cook the pork on medium for about an hour. If you use either a stewing pot or a pressure cooker, you can do the searing in the same pot you'll cook the pork in. Just set aside the meat while you simmer the sauce and then add it back for cooking.

WHAT TO DO

IN A SMALL BOWL, combine the smoked paprika, garlic powder, onion powder, black pepper, salt, and ground coffee to make a spice rub for the pork. Pat the pork dry with a paper towel and generously rub the spices over the three pieces of pork.

IN AN 8-QUART SAUCEPOT, heat the 6 tablespoons of vegetable oil on medium-high until the oil begins to shimmer. Sear each piece of pork, just until brown, on all four sides. If you find the oil is splattering too much, turn the heat down. There's no sense getting burned. Transfer the pork to a Crock-Pot (see tip, page 149).

DISCARD the excess oil, but leave behind any remnants of the meat in the saucepot. Those yummy bits will add flavor to your barbecue sauce.

IN A MEDIUM BOWL, combine the liquor, chicken stock, barbecue sauce, vinegar, brown sugar, and molasses. Whisk well.

WHEN THE SAUCEPOT is no longer hot, add the sauce mixture to the pot. Cook on medium-high and bring the sauce to a boil, taking care to not let the sauce boil over. Pour the sauce over the pork (in the Crock- Pot) and cook on low for 4 hours. (Since the pork is cut into 3 pieces, it won't take as long to cook as a whole 4-pound pork butt would.) Turn off the pot and let the pork rest in the sauce for 30 minutes.

ONCE THE PORK IS DONE, place it on a cutting board and let it rest for 15 minutes.

AS THE LIQUID COOLS, skim the top of it to remove the excess fat. Transfer the liquid to a medium saucepot. Let it simmer until the desired sauce consistency is reached.

WITH TWO FORKS, pull the meat apart until it's all shredded. Discard any excess fat. Add the pork back into the sauce. Simmer for 10 minutes.

SERVE on your favorite bread. I love it on warmed Hawaiian bread or little French rolls. Hamburger rolls are great, too. Garnish with the chopped green onion.

Fresh Cabbage Slaw

SERVES 10 to 12

TOTAL TIME: 15 minutes

This classic is still a great side dish for sandwiches, and I especially like it with the Barbecue Pulled-Pork Sandwiches (page 149).

1 medium green cabbage, shredded (see tip)

1 carrot, peeled and grated

1 medium yellow onion, shaved thin (see tip, page 19)

¼ cup mayonnaise

¼ cup sour cream

6 tablespoons white distilled vinegar (see tip)

¼ cup sugar

1 teaspoon celery seeds

½ teaspoon salt

WHAT TO DO

IN A LARGE BOWL, combine all the ingredients and mix well.

YOU CAN SERVE this right away, but it tastes even better after a few hours in the refrigerator, or even the next day.

the
**BUSY
MOM'S
TIP**

If you don't have white distilled vinegar on hand, you can substitute apple cider vinegar or sherry vinegar.

In a time crunch, you can grab a bag of preshredded cabbage for this dish.

MAKES about 2 quarts
PREP TIME: 10 minutes
(plus 2 hours to rest)

Bread-and-Butter Pickles

It's a good idea to make these pickles ahead of time and store them in the
refrigerator. They need to spend at least two hours in the pickling liquid.
As long as they stay covered in liquid, they'll last for weeks.

6 medium cucumbers with minimal seeds, such as Kirby, Persian, or hothouse

4 cups unseasoned rice vinegar or white distilled vinegar (see tip)

2½ cups sugar

1 teaspoon ground turmeric

1 teaspoon whole mustard seeds

1 teaspoon crushed red pepper flakes

4 big sprigs of fresh tarragon or 1 tablespoon dried tarragon

WHAT TO DO

SLICE the cucumbers into ¼-inch rounds and place them in a large bowl.

IN A MEDIUM SAUCEPAN over high heat, combine the vinegar, sugar, turmeric, mustard seeds, red pepper flakes, and tarragon. As soon as the liquid begins to boil,
remove it from the heat and pour the hot liquid over the cucumber slices.

COVER the bowl with plastic wrap and let it sit in the fridge for 2 hours or overnight.
The pickles can be stored in a clean container for up to 2 weeks. They can be stored
for up to 6 weeks in sanitized mason jars, as long as they're not contaminated by
messy fingers or forks.

Grandma's Lasagna

SERVES 6 to 8
PREP TIME: 45 minutes
COOKING TIME: 40 minutes

I'm really into no-boil, oven-ready lasagna noodles. I'm sure people would expect an Italian chef to insist on fresh pasta, or at least the traditional dried pasta that gets boiled first. But this pasta shaves 15 minutes off your prep time, and you don't lose any quality. Go for the easy stuff!

FOR THE SAUCE

¼ cup olive oil

¼ cup chopped garlic (about 8 cloves)

3 (16-ounce) cans of peeled, whole plum tomatoes (see tip)

½ teaspoon salt

1 teaspoon sugar

FOR THE LASAGNA

¼ cup olive oil

1½ pounds ground turkey (dark or white meat, or a mixture of both)

½ teaspoon salt

2 tablespoons dried Italian seasoning, or 4 teaspoons fresh marjoram
   or oregano

1 (9-ounce) package of no-boil, oven-ready lasagna noodles

Sauce (from above)

½ cup shredded or grated Parmigiano-Reggiano cheese

2 cups whole-milk ricotta cheese

4 cups shredded whole-milk, mozzarella cheese

3 Roma tomatoes, sliced into 6 to 8 slices each (see tip, page 67)

12 medium to large fresh basil leaves

the
**BUSY
MOM'S
TIP**

I prefer San Marzano canned tomatoes. If you can find those, definitely give them a try. They're sweeter than most canned tomatoes and not overly acidic. If you need to use crushed tomatoes, that's okay, too.

WHAT TO DO

FOR THE SAUCE:

HEAT the olive oil in a 4-quart saucepot over medium heat. Add the chopped garlic and just as it starts to brown around the edges, throw in the canned tomatoes. You don't want the garlic to burn, so have the cans open and ready to go beforehand.

ADD the salt and sugar and whisk it all together. Let the sauce simmer on medium-low for 40 minutes while you prep the other ingredients. If any foam rises to the top of the sauce, skim it off. That's the acid from the tomatoes, and your sauce will taste better without it.

USING a hand blender or countertop blender (see tip, page 57), blend on medium until smooth.

FOR THE LASAGNA:

PREHEAT the oven to 375°F.

IN A 10-INCH SAUTÉ PAN, heat the olive oil on medium-high. Add the ground turkey and the salt. Cook the turkey for about 5 minutes, until it's browned throughout. Just as it's finishing the cooking process, stir in the Italian seasoning. Drain any excess fat or liquid from the pan.

COVER the bottom of a 13- x 9-inch baking pan with 3 sheets of pasta. Ladle 1 cup of sauce over the noodles. You don't want the sauce to soak through, so you don't need to overdo it.

LAYER ON HALF OF THE MEAT, followed by half of the Parmigiano-Reggiano, and half of the ricotta cheese. Sprinkle on one-third of the mozzarella and arrange one-third of the fresh tomatoes on top of it. Top with one-third of the basil.

REPEAT the process for the next layer: 3 sheets of pasta, a cup of of sauce, the rest of the meat, the rest of the Parmigiano-Reggiano, the remaining ricotta, a third of the mozzarella, a third of the fresh tomatoes, and another third of the basil.

THE LAST LAYER is your presentation layer, so make it pretty. Add three more sheets of pasta. Top the noodles with the last of the sauce, mozzarella, fresh tomatoes, and basil.

BAKE uncovered for 40 minutes, rotating halfway through. The top should be a crispy golden brown when the lasagna is done, and the pasta sauce around the sides of the dish should be thick, not runny.

LET THE LASAGNA stand for 10 to 15 minutes before serving. If you cut into it while it's still piping hot, it will fall apart.

Old-Fashioned Pot Roast

Whenever you find yourself with half-finished bottles of wine, stick them in the fridge and use them for cooking. There's no point letting them go to waste, and I don't recommend seeking out expensive wines for cooking.

3 pounds boneless chuck roast

¼ cup salt

1 tablespoon black pepper

¼ cup vegetable oil

1 cup all-purpose flour

1 large carrot, peeled and sliced into ½-inch pieces

2 stalks of celery, sliced into ½-inch pieces

1 large yellow onion, sliced ½-inch thick

1 large sprig of fresh rosemary

2 sprigs of fresh thyme

2 tablespoons beef Better Than Bouillon (see tip)

4 cups red wine

3 tablespoons tomato paste

3 tablespoons cornstarch mixed in 3 tablespoons cold water

WHAT TO DO

PREHEAT the oven to 400°F (see tip).

SEASON the roast with the salt and pepper and let it sit for about 5 minutes.

YOU NEED A SHALLOW, 6-quart saucepot that's oven-safe, with an oven-safe lid. In the pot, heat the oil on high.

FLOUR the pot roast with all the flour, shaking off the excess. Sear the pot roast for about 4 minutes on all sides to get a nice brown color. As you turn the roast to the last side, add the carrot, celery, and onion to the pot.

AFTER THE ROAST is seared on all sides, add the rosemary and thyme to the pot. Throw in the bouillon, wine, and tomato paste.

IF THE MEAT isn't quite covered with liquid, add just enough water so that the roast is completely submerged. Cover the pot and turn the heat up to high. Bring the liquid to a boil and transfer the pot to the oven (see tip).

BAKE for 3 hours. Remove the roast from the oven and let it rest in its own juices for 30 minutes. Take the meat out of the pan and set it aside. Strain out the juices into a medium saucepot, setting the veggies aside with the meat. Discard the thyme and rosemary stems.

SIMMER the juices over medium heat. As the oil rises to the top, skim it off, leaving behind the jus. Continue to simmer the jus until you like the taste of it.

ADD the cornstarch-water mixture to the pot. The jus will thicken almost immediately. If it's still too thin for your taste, you can add another batch of the cornstarch-water mixture. If you find it's too thick, you can thin the jus with a bit of water.

SLICE the pot roast and assemble it on a platter with the roasted veggies. Drizzle the jus over all of it and serve.

the
BUSY
MOM'S
TIP

Bringing the liquid to a boil before you transfer the pot to the oven will actually shorten the cooking time, so don't skip that step.

Rosemary Mashed Potatoes

This side dish goes great with the Old-Fashioned Pot Roast (page 156). I prefer to use Yukon Gold potatoes for mashing. Russets are good for making potato salad or hash, and for baking, but are too starchy for mashed potatoes. Yukon Gold potatoes are incredibly flavorful, and they are less starchy and more creamy.

4 medium Gold Yukon potatoes, peeled and cut into sixths (see tip)

4 tablespoons salt (for the boiling water), plus up to 2 teaspoons for the whipped potatoes

1½ cups heavy cream

1 stick (½ cup) unsalted butter, softened

1 tablespoon chopped fresh rosemary

WHAT TO DO

IN A 2-QUART POT, cover the potatoes with cold water. Add 4 tablespoons of salt to the pot and bring the water to a simmer. Simmer for 15 to 20 minutes, until the potatoes are soft.

WHILE THE POTATOES COOK, heat the cream in a small saucepot. Bring it to a simmer and remove from the heat.

DRAIN the water from the potato pot and add the butter to the potatoes.

USE an electric mixer, or an old-fashioned potato masher, to mix the cream into the potatoes while mashing them. Add up to 2 teaspoons of salt if needed. Once the potatoes are mashed, I like to whisk them just to make sure everything is well mixed.

IF YOU WANT EXTRA-SMOOTH MASHED POTATOES, use a rubber spatula to pass them through a fine strainer.

STIR in the fresh rosemary and serve.

---

the
BUSY MOM'S TIP

This is a simple recipe with few ingredients, but what matters most is that the potatoes are cut into equal pieces and that their cooking process starts with cold water. Otherwise, they won't cook at the same speed and you'll end up with lumpy, weird mashed potatoes.

Spaghetti and Meatballs

SERVES 6 to 8
TOTAL TIME: 45 minutes

I cook the meatballs in the oven rather than in the sauce. It's much quicker, and these meatballs are so delicious, you're not sacrificing any flavor. While the sauce simmers, you can get your meatballs prepped and cooking. The most important thing is that you don't overwork them. If you mix them too much, they become too dense—like little golf balls. Instead, put all the ingredients into the bowl and then give it one good mixing. *(see photo insert)*

the BUSY MOM'S TIP

If you prefer a sharper cheese, go with Locatelli, which is a pecorino. Grana Padano is a less expensive version of Parmigiano-Reggiano.

FOR THE SAUCE

¼ cup olive oil

8 garlic cloves, chopped (about ¼ cup)

3 (16-ounce) cans of peeled, whole plum tomatoes (San Marzano are my favorite; see tip, page 153)

½ teaspoon salt

1 teaspoon sugar

FOR THE MEATBALLS

3 slices white bread, crusts removed, cut into ¼-inch cubes

1 cup heavy cream

1 tablespoon unsalted butter

8 garlic cloves, chopped

1 pound ground pork

1 pound ground veal

2 large eggs

½ cup shredded or grated Parmigiano-Reggiano cheese (see tip)

¼ cup chopped fresh marjoram or 2 tablespoons dried marjoram

Dash nutmeg

2 tablespoons salt

2 pounds spaghetti

½ cup shredded or grated Parmigiano-Reggiano cheese, for garnish

¼ cup chopped fresh basil, for garnish

I like to test my meatball mixture before I cook all the meatballs. How else would I know if it's well seasoned? I recommend cooking a small bit of the meatball mixture in a pan with a little oil. If the result isn't flavorful enough, you might need to add more salt.

■

Lately I'm obsessed with perciatelli pasta. It's a thicker spaghetti noodle with a hole running through the center of it. It's hearty enough to stand up to this heavier dish. If you can't find perciatelli, linguine also works well.

WHAT TO DO

PREHEAT the oven to 400°F.

FOR THE SAUCE:

HEAT the olive oil in a 4-quart saucepot over medium heat. Add the chopped garlic, and just as the garlic starts to brown around the edges, throw in the canned tomatoes. You don't want the garlic to burn, so have the cans open and ready to go.

ADD the salt and sugar and whisk it all together. Let the sauce simmer on medium-low for 40 minutes while you prep the other ingredients. If any foam rises to the top of the sauce, skim it off. That's the acid from the tomatoes, and your sauce will taste better without it. Using a hand blender or a countertop blender, blend the sauce on medium until smooth (see tip, page 57).

FOR THE MEATBALLS:

IN A BOWL, cover the bread with the heavy cream and let it sit to absorb the liquid.

IN A SMALL SAUTÉ PAN, heat the butter on medium heat. Add the garlic and cook it just enough to get it warmed through. Remove it from the heat.

PUT THE PORK, veal, sautéed garlic, eggs, Parmigiano-Reggiano, marjoram, nutmeg, and salt in a large bowl. Once the bread has absorbed the cream, add it to the other ingredients. Mix it all with your hands, just until it's well incorporated.

USE a 2-ounce ice cream scoop to measure out equal-sized meatballs. After you've scooped out the proper portions, wet your hands to keep the meat from sticking to them, and roll the meat into ball shapes. Bake the meatballs on a baking sheet for about 15 minutes, until they're springy to the touch.

COOK the pasta according to the package directions. Drain the pasta and add it to the saucepot, covering it with sauce and simmering on medium-low for 2 to 3 minutes. If there's excess water from the pasta noodles, simmer a little longer until the pasta takes on a red color and the sauce thickens.

TO SERVE FAMILY-STYLE, transfer the noodles to a large platter and top with meatballs and sauce. Garnish with Parmigiano-Reggiano and basil.

Escarole Salad

SERVES 4
TOTAL TIME: 10 minutes

I usually serve this salad as an antipasto, or appetizer, before the main course. The fresh white anchovies, also called *boquerónes*, have a much milder, more delicate flavor than most other anchovies.

1 (15.5-ounce) can of white beans

⅓ cup, plus 6 tablespoons extra-virgin olive oil (see tip, page 71)

¼ teaspoon salt

Dash black pepper (just a sprinkle)

1 teaspoon chopped fresh rosemary or ½ teaspoon dried rosemary

2 heads escarole

⅓ cup shaved Parmigiano-Reggiano cheese, plus shreds for garnish (see tip)

⅓ cup Italian flat-leaf parsley leaves

2 tablespoons sherry vinegar or red wine vinegar

4 fresh white anchovies, drained

the BUSY MOM'S TIP

I prefer to buy a block of Parmigiano-Reggiano cheese and shave it with a potato peeler. It's more cost-effective, and the freshly shaved cheese is more flavorful.

WHAT TO DO

DRAIN the beans and combine them in a bowl with the ⅓ cup extra-virgin olive oil, salt, a dash black pepper, and the rosemary. Set the mixture aside to marinate.

REMOVE and discard the green leaves from the outside of the heads of escarole. Chop the hearts into ¼-inch pieces.

IN A LARGE BOWL, combine the escarole, the ⅓ cup Parmigiano-Reggiano, parsley, the 6 tablespoons extra-virgin olive oil, and the vinegar. Toss it all together. Escarole is a hearty green and it will absorb the oil without turning into a wilted mess.

SPRINKLE the beans on top and around the sides of the bowl. Garnish the salad with several shreds of Parmigiano-Reggiano and top with the anchovies.

Crispy Fried Chicken

When I was nineteen years old, I learned how to make fried chicken from a chef in New Orleans. He taught me a great time-saving lesson. With two easy-to-find ingredients—Lawry's seasoned salt and Gulden's spicy brown mustard—you can skip the fancy steps that lots of recipes take before flouring the chicken. Those two ingredients will act as a brine and improve the flavor, texture, and moisture of the meat. *(see photo insert)*

12 to 14 pieces of chicken (legs, thighs, and wings)
5 tablespoons Lawry's seasoned salt
5 tablespoons Gulden's spicy brown mustard or any whole-grain mustard
2 quarts vegetable oil
4 cups all-purpose flour

WHAT TO DO

IN A LARGE BOWL, cover the chicken with the seasoned salt and mustard. Mix it well, so the chicken pieces are coated. Cover the bowl and let the chicken marinate for 10 to 15 minutes, or stick it in the fridge to marinate for up to 6 hours.

IN A DEEP FRYER or a 4-quart saucepot, heat the oil to 325°F, verifying the temperature with a candy thermometer (see tip, page 76).

DUMP the flour in a large resealable ziplock bag. Place 4 pieces of chicken in the bag, seal it, and shake to coat them with flour. Set them aside on a plate. Repeat for all the chicken.

DROP 4 to 5 pieces at a time into the hot oil (see tip), and cook for about 10 minutes. It's super easy to tell when the chicken is done. It floats to the top of the oil.

Work in batches and be careful not to overload the deep fryer or saucepot you're using for frying. If you try to fry too much at once, the temperature of the oil will drop too quickly and you'll end up with soggy, oily chicken. Who wants that?

Smaller pieces, like wings, might be done earlier than the rest. Just go ahead and take them out. Drain the chicken on a paper towel–covered plate.

AS YOU WORK through each batch, make sure you adjust the temperature of the oil to keep it at 325°F. If you find the temperature has dropped, turn the heat up a bit and monitor it.

Warm Mushroom Salad with Poached Eggs and Bacon Vinaigrette

I created this salad for a *Top Chef* sexy salad challenge. What's sexier than breaking into the yolk of a poached egg or eating a salad with flowers? For the greens, I chose mâche, sometimes called lamb's lettuce, because of its velvety texture and mild taste. Along with the luscious poached egg, the meaty texture of the mushrooms makes this a salad that men will enjoy as much as women will. *(see photo insert)*

FOR THE SALAD

1 cup ½-inch diced smoked center-cut bacon

½ cup olive oil

½ cup sunchokes (aka Jerusalem artichokes), peeled and diced in ½-inch pieces

1 pound wild mushrooms (such as maitake, morels, hen of the woods, shimeji, or whatever you can find at your market)

2 teaspoons chopped fresh chervil

2 teaspoons chopped fresh chives

Salt to taste

Black pepper to taste

4 cups mâche (aka lamb's lettuce), or torn butter lettuce

16 squash blossoms, center buds removed

FOR THE VINAIGRETTE

½ cup fat rendered from the chopped bacon (above)

½ cup extra-virgin olive oil

½ cup sherry vinegar

¼ cup Dijon mustard

¼ cup honey

¼ teaspoon salt

¼ teaspoon black pepper

FOR THE POACHED EGGS

6 cups water

½ teaspoon salt

5 tablespoons white distilled vinegar

4 large eggs

WHAT TO DO

FOR THE SALAD:

START with rendering the fat from the bacon. This is a slow-cooking process. If you try to rush it, you'll lose all the rich bacon fat you're trying to render for your dressing and you'll burn the bacon in the process.

ON MEDIUM-LOW HEAT, slowly cook the chopped bacon, so the fat is melted away from the meat. Use an 8-inch pan, so the bacon is crowded in there, and the fat will be easier to preserve. Once the bacon is cooked, strain it and set aside ½ cup bacon fat for the vinaigrette. If you end up with less than ½ cup, you can make up the difference with extra-virgin olive oil. Set aside the bacon.

USE the same pan to sauté the sunchokes. Don't bother cleaning the pan first. Let the sunchokes absorb the flavor of the bacon. Add ¼ cup olive oil to the pan and sauté the sunchokes until they're golden brown and soft. Remove them from the pan and add the remaining ¼ cup olive oil. Sauté the mushrooms until they're cooked through.

IN A LARGE BOWL, mix the mushrooms with the sunchokes, chervil, chives, and bacon. Season the mixture with salt and pepper and set it aside.

FOR THE VINAIGRETTE:

IN A SMALL BOWL, combine the bacon fat and extra-virgin olive oil.

IN A SEPARATE BOWL, combine the sherry vinegar, Dijon mustard, honey, salt, and pepper.

SLOWLY WHISK the oil mixture into the other vinaigrette ingredients. This process should help your dressing blend better than it would if you just threw everything into one bowl. Don't worry if it doesn't blend perfectly. The flavors will still be there.

FOR THE EGGS:

IF YOU'VE NEVER POACHED EGGS, don't just turn the page and look for something easier. It's a simple process, if you know a few tricks.

GET A DEEP SAUCEPOT, 8 to 12 inches round, and fill it with about 6 cups of water. This will allow the eggs plenty of room and make it easy for you to lift them out. Season the water with the salt and add the white vinegar. The acid from the vinegar will help the egg whites congeal around the yolks. (Some people use lemon juice, but I don't like lemon-flavored eggs!) Don't let the water reach a rolling boil. It will break the eggs apart and leave a cloudy mess in your pot.

BREAK 1 egg at a time into a small dish, making sure the yolk isn't broken. Pour each egg into the pot of water. They can all cook at the same time.

THE WATER should be just below a boil, so you see bubbles start to rise to the surface. If you don't have much movement in the water and find that the whites aren't surrounding the yolks, create a bit of movement in the water with your slotted spoon.

LET THE EGGS COOK for 2½ minutes for a soft yolk. If you prefer firm yolks and whites, cook for 7 minutes. Lift the poached eggs from the pot with a slotted spoon.

TO ASSEMBLE

WHILE YOUR EGGS are poaching, combine the mâche and squash blossoms and toss them with all but about 2 tablespoons of the vinaigrette.

ARRANGE the salad on four plates and top with the mushrooms and sunchokes.

LAY a sexy poached egg on top of each salad and drizzle with the remaining vinaigrette.

Bone-in Rib Eye with Sauce

Steak is something that many people think of as a restaurant dish, not something they'll make for themselves. But it's not hard to cook, and having your own individual steak for dinner, in the comfort of your own home, feels like a decadent treat.

FOR THE SAUCE

1 pound beef bones (ask the butcher at your local supermarket)

1⅓ cups peeled and roughly chopped carrots

1⅓ cups roughly chopped celery

1⅓ cups roughly chopped yellow onion (see tip, page 49)

2 bay leaves

4 sprigs of thyme

4 cups brandy

8 cups chicken stock (see tip)

4 cups veal demiglace (see tip)

FOR THE RIB EYES

4 tablespoons oil

4 bone-in rib eyes, 12 to 14 ounces each

4 tablespoons unsalted butter

2 sprigs of fresh thyme, whole

2 garlic cloves, smashed

WHAT TO DO

FOR THE SAUCE:

CARROTS, CELERY, and onions are the common base for this kind of sauce. In French cooking, the combination is referred to as a mirepoix (see tip). Don't waste time trying to beautifully chop the veggies for the sauce. A rough chop will do, since you'll discard them after they've served their purpose in this recipe.

the
**BUSY
MOM'S
TIP**

In a perfect world, we'd all be making our own stock and demiglace at home, but most grocery stores offer nice alternatives that save a lot of time without taking away from the quality of the final product. Brands vary by store, but choose options that are sodium-free or reduced-sodium, so you can stay in control of seasoning the dish. You can also buy the carrots, celery, and onions prechopped and mixed together.

You never want to grill
cold meat. Make sure
you take the rib eyes
out of the fridge 10 to
12 minutes before they
go into the pan. Adding
very cold meat to a
hot pan will bring the
temperature way down
and you'll never get a
good sear on the meat.
Allowing the steaks to
warm closer to room
temperature will make it
easy to get a nice crust
when they hit the pan.

ROAST the beef bones in a large stockpot on high heat until the bones take on a nice caramel color. Add the chopped carrots, celery, and onions and roast until they've browned, about 5 to 8 minutes.

ADD the bay leaves, thyme, brandy, chicken stock, demiglace, and the tomato paste, and let the sauce simmer for 40 minutes.

ADD the chicken stock and veal demiglace and let simmer for about 25 minutes, until the sauce thickens. As it cooks, continually skim off any oil or foam that rises to the top.

STRAIN the sauce into a bowl, using a very fine strainer or a piece of cheesecloth. Return the strained sauce to the pot and let it simmer on low heat, reducing it until it thickens. The goal is to have the sauce cook down to a consistency that will coat the back of the spoon. Reducing decreases the water content and intensifies the flavors.

FOR THE RIB EYES:

ADD 2 tablespoons of the oil to your cold pan to cook the first 2 rib eyes. Your pan should be very, very hot to sear your steaks. Don't be afraid of a hot pan. It's your friend! It will definitely give you a better result (see tip).

WITH YOUR BURNER ON HIGH, as the oil starts to heat up, you'll see it begin to shimmer. You want to see a light smoke escaping from the pan. Heavy smoking is bad.

I LIKE THE RIB eyes cooked medium-rare. Sear the steaks on one side for 4 minutes. Turn them over and let the other side sear for about 30 seconds.

(FOR MEDIUM TO MEDIUM-WELL, preheat the oven to 450°F and cook the steaks in the oven for another 8 minutes. Don't forget to let them rest for 6 minutes when they come out of the oven.)

ADD 2 tablespoons of the butter, the sprigs of thyme, and the smashed garlic clove. The simple addition of the thyme and garlic is an easy way to create more layers of flavor and put a little more love and care into the dish. Let the butter brown, and baste the rib eyes for 3½ minutes. Don't use a turkey baster! That's just dangerous.

Use a metal spoon to scoop the hot butter and continuously pour it over the meat. The meat will reach a lovely golden brown.

MOVE the steaks from the pan onto a platter and pour the browned butter over them. Repeat the process for the other 2 rib eyes.

LET THE STEAKS rest in the butter for about 6 minutes. Discard the thyme and garlic and serve the rib eyes with the sauce.

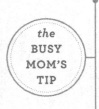

SERVES 4

TOTAL TIME: 15 minutes

the
**BUSY
MOM'S
TIP**

The cipollinis can be cut like an onion. Slice off both ends and cut the cipollinis in half to remove the skin. Slice into quarters.

For this recipe, you're just using the bulbs of the fennel. Cut out the triangular root at the bottom of the bulb. Slice the fennel in half the long way, then slice ¼-inch-thick pieces for this dish. Save the fronds from the fennel and use them to make a fennel mayonnaise for sandwiches.

Roasted Fennel and Cipollini

The savory, licorice flavor of the fennel is perfectly balanced by the wildly sweet taste of the cipollinis, and the dish pairs well with a hearty meat like the Bone-in Rib Eye (page 167). Cipollinis can be found in most supermarkets or farmers' markets, but if you have trouble finding them, you can also substitute shallots or a sweet onion.

½ cup olive oil

2 cups cipollinis, quartered (if substituting an onion, cube into 1-inch pieces; see tip)

¼ teaspoon salt

Dash black pepper

1 tablespoon sugar

4 bulbs fennel, sliced ¼ inch thick (see tip)

WHAT TO DO

ADD half the olive oil to a 10-inch sauté pan and set it on high heat. Once the pan is hot, add the cipollinis, salt, pepper, and the sugar. The sugar will help the cipollinis caramelize, and that's what you want to see happen.

ONCE THE CIPOLLINIS HAVE BROWNED, reduce the temperature to medium and continue sautéing until they soften. Scrape them from the pan and set them aside. Pan-roast the fennel using the same pan and the same process.

ADD the cipollinis back to the pan and combine with the fennel.

the
**BUSY
MOM'S
TIP**

You might be tempted to cook both the fennel and the cipollinis together to save time. Trust me. That's not the right solution. They have different cooking processes and you'll end up with raw cipollinis and mushy fennel. They definitely need to be roasted separately, but you can use the same pan without cleaning it in between.

Shallot-Potato Gratin

I like to serve this decadent side dish with the Bone-In Rib Eye with Sauce (page 167). Don't think about trying to make this a "light" recipe. Embrace the heavy cream! You have all week to worry about how big your butt is or isn't getting. On Sunday night, go ahead and splurge.

2 garlic cloves

4 cups heavy cream

1 sprig of fresh thyme

6 Yukon Gold potatoes, sliced about ¼ inch thick, using a mandoline (see tip page 19)

8 shallots, sliced about ¼ inch thick

Salt to taste

Black pepper to taste

½ cup sour cream

1½ cups shredded whole-milk mozzarella cheese

½ cup panko bread crumbs

WHAT TO DO

HEAT the oven to 350°F.

PUT the garlic cloves on a cutting board and crush them with the flat side of a large knife. Push your weight down on the cloves until they flatten but are still in one piece.

WARMING the cream will prevent the potatoes from discoloring. Pour the cream into a medium pot and add the smashed garlic and thyme. Heat on medium, just until the cream comes to a boil. Take the pot off the heat; use a slotted spoon to remove and discard the cloves of garlic and the sprig of thyme.

IN A 13- X 9-INCH CASSEROLE DISH, layer first the potatoes, then the shallots, followed by just enough cream to cover them. Make sure you season each layer with salt and pepper. Repeat this process until all the potatoes and shallots are used, about 5 layers.

TIGHTLY COVER the dish with foil so no air can escape from it. Bake for 40 to 50 minutes, until the potatoes are cooked through. The potatoes in the center should be soft when you test with a fork.

SPREAD the sour cream over the top of the gratin and layer on the mozzarella cheese. Sprinkle the panko on top and put the uncovered dish under a broiler set to high. Since the food under the broiler can quickly go from brown to burnt, leave the oven door open to remind you to keep an eye on the dish (see tip, page 129). Broil for 3 to 5 minutes, or until the top is golden brown.

Kids in the Kitchen

ITALIAN RICE BALLS

SAMOSAS WITH MANGO SALSA AND CUCUMBER YOGURT SAUCE

TACOS WITH HOMEMADE CORN TORTILLAS

VEGGIE SUSHI ROLLS

CHINESE DUMPLINGS WITH PONZU SAUCE

HOMEMADE LINGUINE

ROASTED ROME APPLES WITH CINNAMON AND CARDAMOM

THE FIRST THING TO KNOW ABOUT GETTING YOUR KIDS INVOLVED IN COOKING: there will be disasters. You just have to live with those moments. Accept that you'll sometimes have a messy kitchen and a little extra cleanup. Someday your kids will tell the story of how you taught them to make their favorite dishes, and you'll see it was all worth it.

I have girlfriends in their thirties who look at a bunch of asparagus in the refrigerator and freak out. They see it as a headache, when it's really a simple vegetable they can have prepped and ready to cook in less than five minutes. It's not their fault. We live in a fast-food world. No one ever taught them how to work with ingredients to create a meal, so they're shy about attempting the simplest things.

As parents, it's our responsibility to give our kids a sense of confidence in the kitchen that will serve them well through adulthood. It's an important life skill, and there's a primal sense of independence from being able to provide your own meal. It's one of the many ways we teach our children to be confident in their ability to take care of themselves.

A few rules for kids in the kitchen:

Kitchen safety is first and foremost. Teach your children to respect kitchen equipment without being afraid of it. Just as the ocean is a fun place to swim and play but can sweep away a careless swimmer, the kitchen is a fun place to experiment and create but can be dangerous if we don't take proper precautions.

Clean as you go. Cooking is a great opportunity to teach kids to be clean and organized while they work. There should always be a sense of organization, purpose, and procedure.

Master the basics. Improvisation is great, but everyone should start by learning basic techniques. It makes the process faster and safer.

Use these easy recipes to spend fun time with your children while giving them a chance to learn skills that will serve them for a lifetime.

Italian Rice Balls

These are a staple in every Italian Long Island family's daily life. They're in every Long Island deli and they're a part of traditional Italian cooking. I've made them every Thanksgiving and Christmas since I was a kid. My mother would set up a little assembly line of ingredients, and I'd do the work. I loved the job. Working with the rice was like playing with Silly Putty.

1 cup arborio rice (risotto rice)

2 cups water

1 tablespoon salt

2 egg yolks

2 cups grated or shredded Parmigiano-Reggiano cheese

¼ cup chopped Italian flat-leaf parsley

¼ cup chopped fresh basil

3 tablespoons chopped sun-dried tomatoes

3 cups vegetable oil

2 cups dried plain bread crumbs

1½ cups cubed firm whole-milk mozzarella cheese (see tip)

WHAT TO DO

IGNORE the directions on the package of rice. In a medium pot, combine the rice, 2 cups water, and the salt and bring to a simmer. Cover the pot and let the rice cook for 12 minutes, or until the water is absorbed.

WHEN THE RICE IS DONE, spread it out on a baking sheet. Use a rubber spatula to move the rice around, allowing the steam to escape and the rice to cool. In a medium bowl, mix the egg yolks and Parmigiano-Reggiano cheese.

ADD the egg-and-cheese mixture, parsley, basil, and sun-dried tomatoes to the cooled rice. Use a rubber spatula to incorporate these ingredients. It will be very sticky. Put the bread crumbs in a medium bowl.

the
BUSY
MOM'S
TIP

Be careful not to buy the semisoft fresh mozzarella you often see in the store. You need to buy a firm block of mozzarella and cut it into cubes. Polly-O is an easy-to-find brand that sells one-pound blocks of mozzarella.

IN A 4-QUART POT, heat the vegetable oil to 350°F, verifying the temperature with a candy thermometer.

SET UP the sheet of rice next to the cheese and the bowl of bread crumbs. The kids will roll the rice balls, but Mom or Dad should handle the frying.

USE a 2-ounce ice cream scoop or a ¼-cup measuring cup to portion out the rice. Roll 1 scoop in your wet hands to shape it into a ball. Push 2 cubes of cheese into the center of the ball. Reshape the rice to close the ball around the cheese. Coat each ball in bread crumbs and set on a plate until ready to fry.

FRY 4 or 5 rice balls at a time for 2 to 3 minutes, until they're golden brown (see tip, page 66). Remove them from the oil with a slotted spoon and set them to drain on a paper towel–lined plate.

IF DESIRED, serve with your favorite marinara sauce or with a homemade sauce like the one I use in Grandma's Lasagna (page 153).

Samosas with Mango Salsa and Cucumber Yogurt Sauce

MAKES 20 samosas
TOTAL TIME: 45 minutes

These are basically Indian dumplings or turnovers. Sometimes stuffed with lamb or beef, they're incredibly common in Indian cuisine. This vegetarian version, stuffed with potatoes and peas, is one of the most popular types of somosa in India and wherever Indian food is enjoyed.

FOR THE SAMOSAS

2 medium russet potatoes, peeled and roughly chopped

1 stick (½ cup) unsalted butter

½ medium yellow onion, diced ¼ inch thick

2 cups frozen peas

2 tablespoons garam masala

1 tablespoon ground cumin

1½ tablespoons salt

2 tablespoons chopped fresh cilantro

2 tablespoons chopped fresh mint

20 wonton wrappers

1 egg yolk mixed with 1 teaspoon cornstarch (This is your glue.)

2 cups vegetable oil

FOR THE MANGO SALSA

1 cup ½-inch-diced mango

½ cup ½-inch-diced hothouse cucumber, skin on

2 tablespoons finely diced red onion

1 tablespoon chopped fresh cilantro

1 tablespoon fresh lime juice

½ teaspoon salt

1 teaspoon sugar

the
BUSY
MOM'S
TIP

A great way to teach your kids about other cultures is through food. Trying different ethnic cuisines is a fun way to bridge school and home.

FOR THE CUCUMBER YOGURT SAUCE

1 cup low-fat plain yogurt

¼ cup shaved hothouse cucumber

1 tablespoon sugar

1 tablespoon fresh lime juice

2 tablespoons chopped fresh mint

WHAT TO DO

FOR THE SAMOSAS:

IN A MEDIUM POT, cover the potatoes with cold water and bring them to a boil. Cook them for 11 to 12 minutes, until they're tender. Drain the potatoes thoroughly. You want to get all the water out of there.

WHILE THE POTATOES COOK, you can start the other vegetables.

IN A 2-QUART SAUCEPOT, melt the butter on medium heat (see tip). Sweat the onion and peas for about 6 minutes, until the onion is very soft.

STIR IN the garam masala and cumin and let them bloom for about 2 minutes. Use a wooden spoon to mix the potatoes with the peas and onions. The potatoes will get partially mashed in the process. Season the mixture with the salt, stirring to make sure it's all well mixed.

POUR the filling into a bowl to let it cool. Add the cilantro and mint.

TO ASSEMBLE EACH SAMOSA, lay out a wonton wrapper. Place a tablespoon of filling in the middle of the wrapper. Brush the edges with the cornstarch mixture, which will act as glue, sealing the edges of the samosa.

THERE ARE SEVERAL DIFFERENT METHODS for folding samosas. A kid-friendly way is to pull the four corners up to meet over the middle. You'll have a round base at the bottom. Close the wrapper by squeezing the four parts together, almost like you're creating a stem on top of the round base. Stick the samosas in the fridge so they'll be cold when you fry them.

IN A 3- TO 4-QUART POT, heat the vegetable oil to 375°F, verifying the temperature with a candy thermometer. Fry four or five samosas at a time for 3 minutes, or until they're golden brown (see tip, page 66). Use a slotted spoon to remove them from the oil and drain on a paper towel–covered plate.

FOR THE MANGO SALSA:

COMBINE the mango, cucumber, onion, cilantro, lime juice, salt, and sugar in a small bowl. Set aside to serve with the samosas.

FOR THE CUCUMBER YOGURT SAUCE:

IN A SMALL BOWL, mix the yogurt, cucumber, sugar, lime juice, and mint. Serve as a dipping sauce for the samosas.

Tacos with Homemade Corn Tortillas

This recipe calls for masa harina, a specially treated, finely ground corn flour. If your local supermarket doesn't have masa harina, check a Mexican specialty store or a high-end grocery store. At some Mexican specialty stores, you can even buy tortilla dough already made and ready to be shaped and cooked. Either way, kids will love the process of working and shaping the dough with their hands.

2 cups masa harina
½ teaspoon baking powder
1½ to 2 cups warm water
Nonstick vegetable oil spray
3 tablespoons vegetable or canola oil
1 pound lean ground sirloin
1 tablespoon ground cumin
½ tablespoon ground coriander
Toppings: finely shredded romaine, cheddar cheese, avocado slices, sour cream, salsa, etc. (optional)

WHAT TO DO

COMBINE the masa and baking powder and add 1½ cups warm water. Knead the mixture to form your dough. If the dough is too dry, gradually add more water until the dough is soft and pliable.

SPRAY an 8- to 12-inch sauté pan lightly with nonstick vegetable oil spray and heat it on medium-high.

SHAPE the masa dough into 16 balls of equal size. Press each ball of dough until it's about ⅛ inch thick (see tip). If the edges of the dough start to crack when it's pressed, add a little water to it.

COOK each tortilla in the sauté pan for about 1 minute on each side. To keep them warm, simply wrap them in a clean dish towel.

IN AN 8-INCH SAUTÉ PAN, heat the vegetable oil on high and add the ground sirloin. Cook for 4 to 5 minutes, until the beef is almost fully cooked, and drain away the excess fat.

RETURN the pan to the heat and add the cumin and coriander. Cook for another 2 minutes.

SERVE the tacos with your family's favorite toppings.

Veggie Sushi Rolls

You'll need a bamboo sushi mat to roll the sushi. You can buy cooked sushi rice from the sushi guy at your supermarket or from a local Japanese restaurant. If you really want to cook the rice yourself, you'll need to use a rice cooker and follow the package directions carefully.

4 nori sheets
4 cups cooked sushi rice
8 thin asparagus spears (see tip)
8 carrot sticks (about 4 inches long by ¼ inch thick)
8 slices avocado
Soy sauce, for serving
Pickled ginger, for serving
Wasabi, for serving

WHAT TO DO

TOAST the nori sheets in a nonstick pan for a minute or two on each side to bring out the flavor of the seaweed. Lay the first sheet on the bamboo mat.

WHEN YOU HANDLE THE SUSHI RICE, your hands need to stay wet or the rice will stick to your fingers. I like to keep a small bowl of water next to me, so I can continuously wet my hands. Just try to avoid wetting the nori sheet.

PLACE 1 cup of rice in the middle of the nori, using your wet fingers to spread it out to cover the sheet completely.

MEASURE about 2 finger-widths up from the edge closest to you. This is where you'll add your vegetables and avocado. Place the 2 asparagus spears with their tips sticking out of the two ends of the roll. Add the carrot sticks and avocado.

If you can find only thick asparagus spears, just blanch them in boiling water for about 2 minutes and shock them in an ice bath to stop the cooking process. The thin asparagus spears can be left raw.

LIFT the edge of the mat closest to you and roll the mat over so that the fillings are covered. The edge of the mat will touch the rice, but that's okay. Pull that first bit of the roll firmly toward you.

RELEASE the mat and lift it over the roll so you can finish rolling the rest of the way, always keeping the mat on top of the nori sheet as you go. Squeeze the mat to make sure the sushi is tightly wrapped.

YOU NEED TO USE a very sharp knife to slice the sushi; otherwise you'll squeeze out the filling. Wet the knife and slice the roll in half (see tip). Serve with soy sauce, pickled ginger, and wasabi.

the BUSY MOM'S TIP

The trick to cutting anything into equal-sized pieces is to continually cut the pieces in half. Rather than working from one end to the other, start in the center.

Chinese Dumplings with Ponzu Sauce

Any combination of white and dark chicken meat will work. If you prefer a leaner option, choose white-meat chicken. Since the recipe includes a sauce, you don't have to worry about the chicken coming out too dry.

For a shrimp dumpling option, omit the chicken from the recipe, and use 1 pound of 11/13-count shrimp, peeled and deveined, and roughly chopped. Defrosted frozen shrimp is fine, but dry it very well before using it. Otherwise the excess liquid will seep through your dumpling wrapper.

Dumplings are very common in Chinese cooking, and they make a perfect comfort food. These can be boiled or fried. If you want to make steamed dumplings, you'll need to visit a specialty store and ask for the wrappers that are made to withstand the steaming process.

FOR THE DUMPLINGS

2 tablespoons canola oil

1 pound ground chicken (see tip)

2 (8-ounce) cans of water chestnuts, drained and roughly chopped

½ cup chopped green onions, including both the green and white parts

¼ cup oyster sauce

20 wonton wrappers

1 egg yolk mixed with 1 teaspoon cornstarch (This is your glue.)

FOR THE PONZU SAUCE

1 cup rice wine vinegar

¼ cup soy sauce

1 tablespoon sugar

2 tablespoons fresh orange juice

½ tablespoon chopped fresh ginger

WHAT TO DO

IN A 10-INCH SAUTÉ PAN, heat the canola oil on medium heat. Let the pan get nice and hot, until the oil shimmers. Add the ground chicken to the pan and sauté it for about 2 minutes, until it's almost done cooking. Stir in the chopped water chestnuts, the green onions, and the oyster sauce. (Oyster sauce is highly seasoned, so you probably won't need more salt.) Taste the chicken. If you feel it needs more salt, you can add some.

TRANSFER the mixture to a bowl and let it cool in the fridge. It should be completely cooled before you start to fill the wrappers.

SCOOP a teaspoon of the filling into the center of a wrapper. Paint the edges of the wrapper with the egg and cornstarch mixture, which will act as a glue to keep the dumpling sealed. Fold the wrapper on a diagonal, forming a triangle. To seal the wrapper, start from one corner and slowly press your way all the way around. You don't want to trap any air inside the dumpling. Repeat until all the wrappers are used. Set the dumplings aside.

BRING a 2-quart pot of water to a boil. Drop in a few dumplings at a time. They'll sink to the bottom, and as soon as they float, they're done. Pull them out with a slotted spoon and drain them on a plate. Don't use paper towels on the plate. They'll just stick to your dumplings. Wipe the plate of excess water instead.

IN A SMALL BOWL, combine the rice wine vinegar, soy sauce, sugar, orange juice, and ginger to make the ponzu sauce (see tip). Serve the dumplings with the sauce for dipping.

the
**BUSY
MOM'S
TIP**

Making a sauce like a ponzu is much better than using soy sauce for dipping. This sauce will have much less sodium than you'd get in a plain soy sauce.

Homemade Linguine

This recipe is fairly easy, but it has a lot of repeated steps and you can expect it to take longer than most. The pasta making takes some time, and it's a very hands-on dish, so read the recipe all the way through before you get started. This rich, delicate noodle is well worth the effort. I like to serve it with the Quick Pasta Sauce (page 71). You can make the sauce while the pasta is resting or while the kids are rolling out the dough.

3 cups all-purpose flour
1 teaspoon salt, plus ¼ cup for boiling the pasta
4 large eggs
2 teaspoons extra-virgin olive oil
2 cups semolina flour, for sprinkling on the rolled pasta

WHAT TO DO

IF YOU HAVE A STAND MIXER, you can just add the pasta ingredients to its bowl and use the kneading attachment to mix and knead the dough. You can also use the pasta roller attachment, but I find rolling out the dough works best with an inexpensive, old-fashioned pasta roller. And it's much more fun for the kids to use, too.

ADD the 3 cups all-purpose flour and 1 teaspoon salt into a large bowl and mix well. Use your hand to create a well in the middle of the mixture. It should be deep enough to hold all the wet ingredients without any of them spilling out.

POUR the eggs and olive oil in the well. Use the tips of your fingers pressed together to make a counterclockwise circular motion through the flour, bringing it into the wet ingredients a little at a time. It will take about 10 minutes to get everything well incorporated, but this process will prevent lumps from forming in the dough.

KNEAD the dough for 3 to 5 minutes.

FORM the dough into a ball and flatten it slightly. It should look like a halfway deflated ball. Cover the dough with plastic and let it rest in the fridge for an hour.

CUT the dough into 6 equal portions and set the pasta attachment on the first setting. You're basically going to knead the dough through a pasta roller (see tip). The trick is in getting the portion of pasta dough to form a rectangular shape. Send the pasta through on the first setting 1 time. Before you send it through again, fold in the sides of the dough, so the two sides meet in the center.

SEND THE PASTA through the roller 3 more times on the first setting. After each pass, fold in the sides, so that you get a more rectangular shape. This is a great job for the kids!

NOW THE PASTA NEEDS to go through the roller 1 time on each setting, working through setting number 5, but you don't have to fold the sides anymore, and it only needs to go through each level one time. Don't try to skip any settings. It won't work out well.

REPEAT the process for the remaining portions of pasta. Yes, this takes some time, but it's so worth it. Hold all the sheets of pasta on a baking sheet or countertop dusted with semolina.

ONCE ALL THE PASTA has been rolled flat, cut it into sheets about 8 to 10 inches long.

CHANGE THE SETTING on the roller to make linguine noodles. Feed the pasta through to cut it into the noodles.

AS EACH BATCH OF NOODLES is made, hold the noodles over a sheet of parchment paper and sprinkle them with semolina, so they won't stick together. As you work through the batches, keep the pasta in the fridge so it doesn't get too warm or too mushy. Just lay it out on a baking sheet covered with parchment paper generously dusted with semolina flour. Don't worry if the noodles overlap (see tip).

FILL an 8-quart saucepot halfway with water. Add ¼ cup salt to the pot, and bring the water to a rolling boil. The movement will keep the pasta from sticking.

the BUSY MOM'S TIP

If you and your family enjoy the pasta-making process, consider investing in a pasta-drying rack. They're super inexpensive and you can use it to hold the sheets of pasta dough as you work. In the meantime, clear your countertops off completely to have workspace for pasta making.

BEFORE YOU DROP the pasta in the boiling water, make sure your sauce is done and you're ready to eat. Fresh pasta waits for no one.

ADD the fresh pasta into the boiling water and stir it so it doesn't stick together. Cook the pasta for 3 to 4 minutes, until it floats to the top of the water.

DRAIN the pasta and serve immediately with your favorite pasta sauce.

Roasted Rome Apples with Cinnamon and Cardamom

SERVES 4
PREP TIME: 10 minutes
COOKING TIME:
1½ hours

When I was a kid, my mom would help us make these apples. It was her way of teaching us that a fairly healthy dessert can be just as delicious as cookies or cake. Younger children may need help coring the apples, but with a little supervision, they can do the rest of this recipe on their own.

4 Rome Beauty apples (see tip)

½ cup sugar

1 teaspoon nutmeg

¼ teaspoon ground cardamom

¼ teaspoon ground cloves

¼ teaspoon salt

4 cinnamon sticks

2 cups water

Ice cream of your choice, for serving

WHAT TO DO

PREHEAT the oven to 375°F.

CORE the apples and set them in a small oven-safe glass pan.

IN A SMALL BOWL, mix the sugar, nutmeg, cardamom, cloves, and salt. Keeping the apples over the pan, rub the dry mix on the inside and outside of the apples. Allow the excess mixture to fall into the pan.

PLACE one cinnamon stick in the center of each apple. Pour the water into the pan and cover the pan with foil.

BAKE for 1½ hours. When the tops of the apples begin to split, they're done.

LET COOL, then serve with your favorite ice cream.

the
BUSY MOM'S TIP

Rome Beauty apples are available in most areas only during the winter, but they really are the best choice for this dish. I don't recommend any substitutions.

Sweetness

FRUIT SOUP

STRAWBERRY SHORTCAKES WITH WHIPPED CREAM

PEACH BUNDT CAKE

OREO COOKIE ICE CREAM

SPICED CHOCOLATE PUDDING WITH SALTED WHIPPED CREAM

DEEP-FRIED FLUFFER NUTTER SANDWHICH

CHOCOLATE-BANANA-CARAMEL BREAD PUDDING

MY FAMILY LIFE REVOLVED AROUND FOOD AS I GREW UP, AND IT WAS ALWAYS the women who did the cooking. It was just expected that a woman in a traditional Italian family would know how to cook. The men sat around talking while we made them eight-course meals.

So, I grew up cooking, but until I started going to dinner at friends' houses, the only kind of food I was familiar with was Italian food. Once I ventured out of our family kitchen, I was amazed by the whole American genre of food. There was pot roast, tuna casserole, fried chicken, and all kinds of things I'd never eaten at home. One day, a friend's mom brought out a Jell-O mold with fruit floating in it, and the idea of it blew me away. It was so different from the cannoli, Italian wedding cookies, and tiramisù I was used to having for dessert.

My childhood obsession with gelatin was born. I made a new twist on the Jell-O mold every single day for months. Night after night, I presented it to my family for dessert, as if it was the greatest culinary achievement the world had seen. My dad eventually got sick of Jell-O and made me stop, but I had gotten my first taste of experimenting with cuisines outside of the one I grew up with. Cooking became my main creative outlet, and it still is, of course.

There are no Jell-O recipes in this chapter, but I've included everything from cakes to pudding and ice cream. I hope you and your family will find something here that will inspire you as much as that classically American dessert inspired me as a kid.

Fruit Soup

This recipe was inspired by a late-night snack my mom used to make for my brother and me when we were kids. When my dad worked late, we'd crawl in their bed and eat cantaloupe and ice cream. My dad would come home to find us sprawled out fast asleep, and he'd have to carry us to our bedrooms. Inspired by that memory, I like to make this dish to remind my daughter that dessert can also mean fruit.

1 cup water
½ cup sugar
4 cups assorted fruit, chopped in 1- or 2-inch pieces
4 butter wafer cookies
4 scoops vanilla ice cream

WHAT TO DO

A TRADITIONAL SIMPLE SYRUP is equal parts sugar and water. This is a reduced-sugar version. In a medium saucepot, bring the water and sugar to a boil over high heat to create the syrup. As soon as it boils, remove the pot from the heat.

POUR the syrup over the chopped fruit in a large bowl.

SCOOP 1 cup of fruit and liquid into 4 serving dishes. Lay a cookie on top of the fruit. Add a scoop of vanilla ice cream and serve.

---

the
**BUSY
MOM'S
TIP**

My favorite fruits for this dish are cantaloupe, grapes, strawberries, pineapple, and orange segments. If clementines, mandarin oranges, or tangelos are in season, they make a perfect addition, and you can just peel them and pull them apart.

For homemade vanilla ice cream, simply omit the cookies from the Oreo Cookie Ice Cream (page 198).

Strawberry Shortcakes with Whipped Cream

Strawberry shortcake is always a favorite, but you can use a combination of any berries you like for this recipe. *(see photo insert)*

FOR THE SHORTCAKE BISCUITS

1½ cups sliced strawberries

2 tablespoons fresh lemon juice

¼ cup sugar, plus ¼ cup for the biscuits

1½ cups all-purpose flour, plus more for rolling

1 tablespoon baking powder

1 teaspoon salt

¼ teaspoon nutmeg

¼ teaspoon ground cinnamon

1 stick (½ cup) cold unsalted butter, cubed

¼ cup heavy cream

2 large eggs

FOR THE WHIPPED CREAM

2 cups heavy cream

¼ cup powdered sugar, plus more for garnish (optional)

1 teaspoon vanilla

WHAT TO DO

FOR THE SHORTCAKE BISCUITS:

PREHEAT the oven to 375°F.

IN A MEDIUM BOWL, combine the strawberries with the lemon juice and ¼ cup of the sugar. Set aside.

IN A LARGE BOWL, combine the flour, the remaining ¼ cup sugar, and the baking powder, salt, nutmeg, and cinnamon. Pinch the cold butter into the dry ingredients with your fingers for 3 to 4 minutes, until it becomes crumbly. You can also use a couple of spoons for this process.

ONCE THE BUTTER IS INCORPORATED into the dry ingredients, mix the ¼ cup heavy cream and 1 egg together, then add the mixture to the dry ingredients. Knead the dough for about 2 minutes.

ON A LIGHTLY FLOURED WORKSPACE, using a lightly floured rolling pin, roll out the dough until it's 1½ inches thick. For a round shape, you can use a 6-inch cookie cutter to cut out the biscuits (see tip, page 22). If you prefer squares, simply use a knife to cut out 6 biscuits.

BEAT the remaining egg, and use a pastry brush to paint the tops of the biscuits with the egg.

ARRANGE the biscuits on a baking sheet and bake for 12 to 14 minutes. The tops should be golden brown and firm to the touch.

FOR THE WHIPPED CREAM:
IN A LARGE BOWL, combine the 2 cups heavy cream, powdered sugar, and vanilla. Your goal is to make stiff peaks of cream. This means that you'll whip the cream a little longer than usual. That way it'll be firm enough to support the top of the biscuit. You can use a whisk to beat the cream mixture by hand, but it will take about 10 minutes. A hand mixer on high speed will cut that time in half. Whip until the cream forms stiff peaks.

TO ASSEMBLE

Once the biscuits have cooled completely, slice them in half, as if for sandwiches. Top each biscuit base with 3 or 4 spoonfuls of whipped cream. Add 5 or 6 strawberry slices and cover with the biscuit tops. Garnish with powdered sugar, if desired.

Peach Bundt Cake

If you have fresh peaches, they'll work great in this cake. Just make sure they're peeled. Frozen fruit won't work, because the water content is too high.

2 sticks (1 cup) unsalted butter, softened

2 cups sugar

4 large eggs

1 tablespoon vanilla extract

1 (16-ounce) can of sliced peaches, drained of juices and roughly chopped

3 cups all-purpose flour (see tip)

1 teaspoon salt

1½ teaspoons baking powder

¼ cup buttermilk or whole milk

Nonstick vegetable oil spray

WHAT TO DO

PREHEAT oven to 350°F.

WITH A HAND MIXER on high speed or a stand mixer with a paddle attachment, beat the butter and sugar for about 5 minutes, until the mixture is light and fluffy. It should look like whipped cream in texture and color. As you're beating, scrape the sides of the bowl with a rubber spatula to make sure all of the butter is incorporated.

ADD the eggs one at a time while continuing to beat on high (see tip). Add the vanilla and beat the mixture on high speed for another 4 to 5 minutes, scraping the sides of the bowl as you beat.

IN A MEDIUM BOWL, toss the peaches with ¼ cup of the flour, coating the fruit. Add the peach-and-flour mixture to your mixing bowl and beat on high until the peaches are incorporated.

---

the BUSY MOM'S TIP

A portion of the flour will be used to coat the peaches before they're added to the cake batter. This will prevent the fruit from sinking to the bottom of the cake pan.

■

Crack each egg into a small bowl before adding it to the batter. That way, you can remove any shells or get rid of a bad egg without ruining your mixture.

196

IN A SEPARATE BOWL, combine the remaining 2¾ cups flour with the salt and baking powder.

TURN the hand mixer down to a low speed. Add about half of the dry ingredients, taking care to scrape the sides of the bowl to make sure all the ingredients are well blended. Add the buttermilk and continue to mix. Finish by adding the rest of the dry ingredients and incorporating it into the batter.

SPRAY a nonstick Bundt pan with nonstick vegetable oil spray. Pour in the cake batter and bake for 50 to 55 minutes. A toothpick or knife inserted into the cake center should come out dry. If it's wet, let the cake bake a few more minutes.

REMOVE the pan from the oven and let the cake cool for 15 minutes. Flip it onto a plate to serve.

Oreo Cookie Ice Cream

The ice cream base in this recipe can also be used as a warm vanilla sauce to serve over fruit, cake, or even ice cream. The same sauce is used in the Chocolate-Banana-Caramel Bread Pudding (page 204).

You'll need an ice cream machine to make ice cream, but they're inexpensive and worth the small investment. I like the Cuisinart, but there are others that are even less expensive and still get the job done. The machines come with a base that needs to be frozen. I suggest keeping it in the freezer all the time, so you can make ice cream whenever you want.

4 cups heavy cream

1 tablespoon vanilla extract or the seeds scraped from 1 vanilla bean

9 egg yolks

1½ cups sugar

1 cup crushed Oreo cookies

WHAT TO DO

IN A 2- TO 3-QUART SAUCEPOT, heat the cream and vanilla on medium heat. Don't bring it to a boil. You want to scald the cream—simply warm it until a film forms on the top. It should take about 5 minutes.

WHILE THE CREAM IS SCALDING, whisk the egg yolks with the sugar for about 5 minutes, until they're white and frothy. This process will cure the yolks slightly and prevent them from separating. To keep the bowl in place while you whisk, shape a dish towel in a circle on the countertop and place the bowl in the center of it.

ONCE THE CREAM IS READY, remove it from the heat and stir it to allow some of the heat to escape. To prevent the yolks from curdling, you need to add just a little of the hot cream mixture at a time. This is called tempering the yokes. Ladle about ¼ cup of the hot cream into the eggs, whisking so the eggs don't cook under the hot mixture. Add another ¼ cup of the hot cream and whisk it into the eggs. Finally, whisk in the rest of the hot cream.

POUR the mixture back into the saucepot and heat it on medium-low while con-

198

tinuously stirring with a wooden spoon or rubber spatula. Use the spoon or spatula to create figure eights in the pot. This movement will create a whirlpool effect and prevent the coagulation of the eggs. Continue cooking for 4 to 5 minutes. This is your ice cream base and it needs to be babysat while it's on the stove. Have a large bowl ready to pour the base into as soon as it's ready.

AS THE BASE COOKS, it will thicken. You'll know it's ready when it goes from a watery mixture to a consistency thick enough to coat the back of your spoon or spatula really well. At this point, it can easily curdle, so immediately remove it from the heat.

POUR the base into a large bowl and place it in the fridge to cool for 15 to 20 minutes. If you want to speed the cooling, you can place the bowl on top of a bowl of ice and stir to let the heat escape.

ONCE THE BASE IS COOLED, follow the instructions for your ice cream machine. The process should take about 15 minutes. As you near the last few minutes, add the crushed Oreos to the ice cream.

Spiced Chocolate Pudding with Salted Whipped Cream

the
BUSY MOM'S TIP

Whatever small fruit that's in season can be used to top this pudding (with the exception of citrus). I like to use berries or pomegranates.

I make this spicy, sweet, and salty pudding in my restaurant, and it's incredibly popular. Luckily, it's also easy to make. You can even prepare it a couple of days in advance of when you plan to serve it.

FOR THE PUDDING

*2 dried ancho chile peppers, chopped with seeds, or 1 teaspoon
    ancho chile powder*

2 cups heavy cream

2 cups whole milk

1 cup sugar

½ cup cocoa powder

Pinch of crushed red pepper (about ¼ teaspoon)

4 egg yolks

⅓ cup cornstarch

FOR THE SALTED WHIPPED CREAM

2 cups heavy cream

1 tablespoon salt

fruit, for garnish (see tip)

WHAT TO DO

FOR THE PUDDING:

PREHEAT the oven to 500°F (see tip, page 91).

STICK the ancho chile peppers in the oven for about 5 minutes, just to get them nice and toasty. (If you're using ancho chile powder, skip this step.)

IN A 2-QUART POT over medium heat, combine the chile peppers, cream, milk, sugar, cocoa powder, and red pepper and bring it to a scald. You don't want to bring it to a boil. Just heat it until a film forms on top of the liquid.

IN A LARGE MIXING BOWL, combine the egg yolks with the cornstarch.

THE HOT LIQUID needs to be added to the eggs, but you'll temper the eggs to prevent them from curdling. Whisk in only ¼ cup of the hot cream mixture. Repeat the procedure 3 times, then pour in the rest of the mixture.

POUR it all back into the saucepot and heat on medium-low while stirring with a whisk or spatula so the bottom doesn't scald. Cook for 3 to 4 minutes. The mixture will come together and begin to thicken (enough to coat the back of a spoon) and it will continue to thicken to a pudding consistency as it cools.

STRAIN the mixture to discard the chile peppers.

POUR the mixture into a large bowl, or into individual serving bowls, and put it in the fridge to cool. You can even serve it warm if you prefer, but serve the whipped cream on the side, so it doesn't melt.

FOR THE SALTED WHIPPED CREAM:

COMBINE the heavy cream and salt in a large bowl. You can beat it by hand with a whisk for about 8 minutes, or use a hand mixer on high speed for 2 to 3 minutes, until medium peaks form.

TOP the pudding with whipped cream, garnish with fruit, and serve.

Deep-Fried Fluffer Nutter Sandwich

When I was a kid, my mom was big on serving her family real foods. She never let me have fun foods like Marshmallow Fluff, and I was always trying to sneak over to my friend's house, where they had all the good stuff. Now this Marshmallow Fluff dessert is my restaurant's best seller. People come in and take pictures of it, blog about it, and come back for more. Sorry, Mom!

2 cups vegetable oil

2 slices bread (see tip)

3 tablespoons peanut butter

¼ medium banana, thinly sliced

5 tablespoons COLD Marshmallow Fluff

⅓ cup all-purpose flour

2 large eggs, beaten

½ cup panko bread crumbs

Dash salt

WHAT TO DO

IN A 10- TO 12-INCH SAUTÉ PAN, heat the oil to 350°F, verifying the temperature with a candy thermometer (see tip, page 76). The oil needs to be hot and ready to go before the sandwich is made.

WHILE THE OIL HEATS, spread the peanut butter on 1 slice of bread and top it with the banana.

SPREAD the Marshmallow Fluff on the other slice of bread, and put your sandwich together.

PUT the flour, eggs, and panko in three separate bowls big enough for the sandwich.

I like to use pain de mie or brioche, but challah also works well, and even good old white bread will do.

When you flour the sandwich, make sure you cover every bit of it, especially any oozing Marshmallow Fluff. Otherwise the fluff will spew all over the pan.

DUST the entire sandwich in flour (see tip, page 202). Dredge it in the eggs and, with a dry hand, coat it in the panko.

PLACE the sandwich in the oil, and fry it for about 2 minutes, or until that side is golden brown. Use two forks to flip the sandwich, and fry the other side until it's golden brown, too.

WITH A SPATULA, move the sandwich from the pan to a plate. Sprinkle it with the salt, slice it in half, and serve.

the
BUSY
MOM'S
TIP

The caramel sauce is
hands-off when it's
cooking. Once you
dissolve the sugar with
the water, you don't want
to stir or touch the sugar
until it's browned. Don't
try to taste it either. It's
like molten lava. It'll melt
the skin off your finger.

Chocolate-Banana-Caramel Bread Pudding

I've included directions to make a caramel sauce at home. It's easy to make, but the store-bought caramel sauces are just as good, so choose whichever works for you.

FOR THE VANILLA SAUCE

8 cups heavy cream

2 tablespoons vanilla extract or the seeds scraped from 2 vanilla beans

14 egg yolks

1½ cups sugar

FOR THE BREAD PUDDING

1 large baguette, cut into 1-inch cubes (about 8 cups)

1 cup bittersweet chocolate chips

4 medium bananas, sliced in 1½-inch pieces

Vanilla sauce (from above)

1 (12-ounce) jar caramel sauce or homemade caramel sauce (from below)

FOR THE CARAMEL SAUCE

1 cup sugar

2 tablespoons water

½ cup heavy cream, at room temperature

WHAT TO DO

PREHEAT the oven to 375°F.

FOR THE VANILLA SAUCE:

IN A 4- TO 6-QUART SAUCEPOT, heat the cream and vanilla over medium heat. Don't bring it to a boil. You want to scald the cream—simply warm it until a film forms on the top. It should take about 5 minutes.

WHILE THE CREAM IS SCALDING, beat the egg yolks with the sugar for about 5 minutes, until they're white and frothy. This process will cure the yolks slightly.

ONCE THE CREAM IS READY, remove it from the heat and stir it to allow some of the heat to escape. To prevent the yolks from curdling, you need to add a little of the hot cream mixture at a time. This is called tempering the egg yolks. Ladle about ¼ cup of the hot cream into the eggs, whisking so the eggs don't cook under the hot liquid. Add another ¼ cup of the hot cream and whisk it into the eggs. Finally, whisk in the rest of the cream.

POUR the mixture back into the saucepot and heat it on medium-low while continuously stirring with a wooden spoon or rubber spatula. Use the spoon or spatula to create figure eights in the pot. This movement will create a whirlpool effect and prevent the coagulation of the eggs. Continue cooking for 4 to 5 minutes. As the sauce cooks, it will thicken. You'll know it's ready when it goes from a watery mixture to being thick enough to coat the back of your spoon or spatula really well.

FOR THE BREAD PUDDING:

PLACE the bread in the bottom of a 12- x 14-inch baking dish. Sprinkle on the chocolate chips, moving the bread around to allow the chips to get between bread pieces without tossing them all to the bottom of the pan.

INSERT the banana slices between the pieces of bread.

POUR 6 cups of the vanilla sauce over the bread, chocolate chips, and bananas. Bake for 40 minutes. It should be a bit crispy on the top and firm to touch. Remove the pudding from the oven and let it sit for 10 minutes.

FOR THE CARAMEL SAUCE:

IN A 1- TO 2-QUART SAUCEPAN, combine the sugar and water and heat without stirring on medium for about 5 minutes. The sugar will turn from white granulated sugar to light brown melted sugar (see tip, page 204).

IF THERE ARE SUGAR CRYSTALS sticking to the sides of the pan, use a wet pastry brush to dissolve them and gently brush them back to the bottom.

ONCE THE SUGAR HAS BROWNED, turn the heat down to low and slowly stir in the heavy cream. Continue to stir until the mixture forms a sauce.

TO SERVE

SPOON the caramel over the bread pudding. Serve family-style, with the remaining vanilla sauce on the side.

ACKNOWLEDGMENTS

Writing a book and getting it into readers' hands is such a team effort. I'm filled with gratitude for everyone who helped me to bring this from the idea stage to this finished project.

The viewers who cheered for me as I competed on *Top Chef,* and every fan of my food, provided the inspiration to make this book as reader-friendly as possible. Without their interest and support, there'd be no need for this project.

My cowriter, Candice Davis, and her family have been along for this ride since the early stages. They've demonstrated faith in my talent, had patience with my crazy schedule, and turned their family kitchen into a test kitchen for my recipes.

Michael Psaltis has been a phenomenal literary agent. I'd almost swear I heard a hint of excitement in his voice when we finally struck a deal.

Lucia Watson and the team at Penguin believed in *The Busy Mom's Cookbook* and saw the value in it from the beginning, and throughout the writing process they helped me to shape it into the best book it could be. Gabrielle Campo brought a sharp eye for detail to these pages.

Hubert Keller, Anthony Bourdain, and Carla Hall are three amazing chefs who believed in this project and gave voice to their support.

Hayley Lozitsky started this entire process and helped me get to the heart of what this book should be about, no small feat with everything I had going on. Not only did she believe in my talent enough to become my first agent, she continues to be a good friend.

The team at Bullfrog & Baum has been a loyal and constant source of encouragement. Cameron Levkoff seems to always know what I need, and Susan Hosmer offers unconditional support.

Ryan Hayden and the folks at UTA recognized the value in this project and offered their support.

Attorneys Michael Wolf and Neil Tabachnick have provided a steady and consistent presence, always taking care of me through this process.

Wolfgang Puck, Lee Hefter, Thomas Boyce, Ari Rosenson, and David McIntyre, my chef mentors at Spago, taught me so much about cooking and consistently supported my passion for food. These guys make our industry a better place.

Sal Aurora and Mario Guddemi, along with everyone at Black Market, have supported me and encouraged me in all of my endeavors. Gema Martinez has worked tirelessly as my sous chef and pulled two round-the-clock days of cooking to get the food photos done.

Ellen and John Vein generously opened their home to me for the cover photo shoot.

I can always count on Lina Priest to clean me up and take care of the dark circles under my eyes when I'm working too much. Her skill with hair and makeup is the only reason I looked presentable for the cover shoot.

Louise Leonard is a great friend and an amazing food stylist. Because of her talent and professionalism, I was able to trust that the food photos would serve to inspire the reader to get in the kitchen and cook.

Alex Martinez took the amazing pictures of my food (along with his assistant Aubrey Longley-Cook), and Julie Toy shot the cover photo. The photos add a bit of something every cookbook needs—visual flavor.

The Myers family has supported me from the beginning of my journey as a mom and as a chef, and they continue to be a source of encouragement.

Leyla Jacobson, Laura Merians, and Lara Alameh have truly been, and continue to be, lifelong friends. My girls have celebrated all my wonderful firsts with me, including the writing and publication of this book.

Both of my grandmothers inspired me so much. While one made me potato latkes and brisket, the other made pasta and broccoli. They'd both be so proud to see their heritage shared with so many people.

Aunt Annie was one of the women who taught me how to cook when I was growing up. I can't figure out why she thinks she needs my advice about food just because I'm a professional chef.

My brother Dominick, my best friend and confidante, takes kitchen creativity to a whole different level. More importantly, no matter what I say or do, I can trust he'll be there for me without judgment.

My brother Anthony is a constant source of peace and innocence. His presence in the family keeps us all connected and reminds his older siblings to come home.

No matter what I set out to do, my mother always encourages my efforts. She never lets me forget that "Somewhere over the rainbow, dreams really do come true."

From my happiest days to my most heartbreaking moments, I can always count on my dad to be there. I just look to my left or look to my right, and I know I'll find him by my side.

Xea's father, Dwight Myers, not only helped me to create a family, but also inspired me to make a career of what I love to do and to completely commit to it at a very young age. I will forever be grateful.

Lastly, I'd like to thank God for the many blessings I receive each and every day.

INDEX